Praise for *The Dysautonomia Project*

Dysautonomia, which includes POTS, has been increasingly diagnosed over the last few years as an independent medical condition, which also coexists with other conditions, including bladder pain syndrome/interstitial cystitis, chronic fatigue syndrome, Ehlers-Danlos syndrome, fibromyalgia syndrome, Gulf War syndrome, mastocytosis and more. However, there has never been a comprehensive volume addressing dysautonomia diagnosis, pathophysiology and treatment approaches. *The Dysautonomia Project* is a laudable effort to bring the available information together in an organized and easy-to-read fashion.

Theoharis C. Theoharides, PhD, MD, FAAAAI
Tufts University School of Medicine, Boston, MA

This book is a gift to the dysautonomia community. It tells patients who are struggling to understand what's wrong with them that they're not crazy, depressed, or calling out for attention. It helps primary care physicians to become informed enough about the autonomic nervous system to quickly diagnose and refer patients to the right subspecialists and toward symptom relief. For both, it demystifies a condition that disables too many people for too long and disrupts too many lives.

Deborah J. Cornwall, Author
www.thingsiwishidknown.com

As a mom, when your child is sick it feels like your world is upside down. You start feeling overwhelmed, powerless, isolated, and confused. This book will help you to understand the complexity of the autonomic nervous system, dysautonomia, and other co-existing disorders. It will help you understand your child's symptoms and open up dialogue with your doctors. Easy to read and comprehend, it will help you navigate the complex world of autonomic disorders so you can learn the right questions to ask, get the best treatments, and be empowered to become a partner in improving health.

Myrna Concepcion, Mother
Lutz, FL

This is a huge and amazing project! I still remember Doctor Phil Fischer's response to me when my daughter, Michelle, was diagnosed with POTS in 2010. I asked him, "If I were to line up 100 physicians in Spokane, Washington and asked each if they had ever heard of POTS, how many would respond in the affirmative?" He said, "Maybe one!" Now, nearly six years later, if we can get those same 100 physicians to invest in the education that The Dysautonomia Project provides, that "one" would easily turn into 99!" I believe this book will be the resource for the future standard of care for all those patients and families that are impacted by dysautonomia!

Blake Nelson, RPh, MBA, Father
Spokane, Washington

We were one of the lucky ones— for my daughter it took only a little over two years from onset to diagnosis. It was, however, the longest, scariest and most devastating two years of our lives. As we moved from one misdiagnosis to another, spanning from anorexia to cancer to "she's too pretty to be sick," I begged each and every doctor to look at the whole person! It wasn't just her stomach or her throat or her head. It wasn't just a coincidence and bad luck that she was "catching" every germ that flew by. I am elated that *The Dysautonomia Project* is empowering patients and parents with this valuable resource to bridge the gap and provide this much needed information for all practitioners who will undoubtedly use this tool to recognize dysautonomia.

Lisa Rooker, Mother
Tarpon Springs, FL

The Dysautonomia Project

for Patients and Physicians

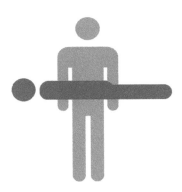

Kelly Freeman, MSM
David S. Goldstein, MD, PhD
Charles R. Thompson, MD

Foreword by David Robertson, MD

Bardolf & Company

THE DYSAUTONOMIA PROJECT
  Understanding Autonomic Nervous System Disorders
  for Physicians and Patients

ISBN 978-1-938842-24-5

Copyright © 2015 by Kelly Freeman, David S. Goldstein,
  and Charles R. Thompson

  Published by Bardolf & Company
  5430 Colewood Pl
  Sarasota, FL 34232
  941-232-0113
  www.bardolfandcompany.com

Cover design by Shaw Creative
www.shawcreativegroup.com

This book is dedicated to the memory of
Cecil Coghlan, MD (1931-2014).
After a 50-year career in cardiology,
he retired as a professor Emeritus
in the division of Cardiovascular Disease
at the University of Alabama in Birmingham.

He was the smartest person I have ever encountered. But he was also, meek, humble, and made you feel like you were the most important person he saw that day. If not for him, most of us with dysautonomia would probably still be undiagnosed. We lost not just a great doctor, but an even better human being.

Randy Thompson, MD

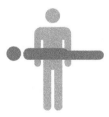

This book is also dedicated
to the millions of undiagnosed patients
with dysautonomia today.

Table of Contents

THE DYSAUTONOMIA PROJECT

The Dysautonomia Project is a not-for-profit collaborative effort of hundreds of volunteer physicians, patients, and community leaders. Our aim is to bridge the wide knowledge gap between community-based physicians and decades of validated clinical research about dysautonomia.

Dysautonomia (Dis-auto-NO-mia) is a general term used to describe any disorder of the autonomic (or automatic nervous) system. These disorders usually involve abnormal symptoms in many organ systems, including cardiac, gastrointestinal, neurological, and pulmonary, as well as others.

The biggest problem in autonomic medicine today is the lack of knowledge about dysautonomia in communities, and especially community-based physicians across the globe because:

- It is not rare, but it is rarely known;
- It changes how every clinician, in every specialty, should approach assessment and treatment of this patient population;
- Every physician, often without knowing it, has at least a handful of dysautonomia patients under his or her care.

The project was launched in the metropolitan area of Tampa Bay, Florida in October 2014, and is currently expanding into communities across the nation and the world.

Dysautonomia, an invisible illness, may be one of the most misdiagnosed medical conditions of all time. Although many decades of clinical research predate this project, disorders of the autonomic nervous system are not taught well, and in some cases completely absent in medical education today.

This book is written by physicians & patients *for* physicians & patients. We hope this book helps facilitate more meaningful discussions in clinic and hospital settings, and speeds the time to proper assessment and treatment of patients with dysautonomia. We invite you to join The Dysautonomia Project and collaborate with us to transform health care for dysautonomia patients around the world.

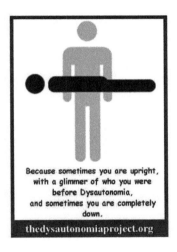

Our logo was designed by the teenage daughter of The Dysautonomia Project *founder. She would witness her mom be able to look normal one day and be completely bedridden the next...leading to the logo of two figures—one upright and the other prone.*

MEDICAL DISCLAIMER

The information and contents, including medical information, in this book are strictly offered as an educational and informational resource only. The Dysautonomia Project book's use shall be expressly limited as an informational tool to help improve awareness and understanding of dysautonomia for both patients and physicians. This book is not intended to and does not provide medical or professional advice or diagnosis, medical or professional opinion, or medical or professional treatment services of any kind to any individual. This book shall in no way substitute or replace a patient-physician relationship or be used as a substitute for medical or professional diagnosis and treatment. Please consult a board certified physician for medical advice or treatment and before making any decisions or changes in your healthcare treatment plan(s).

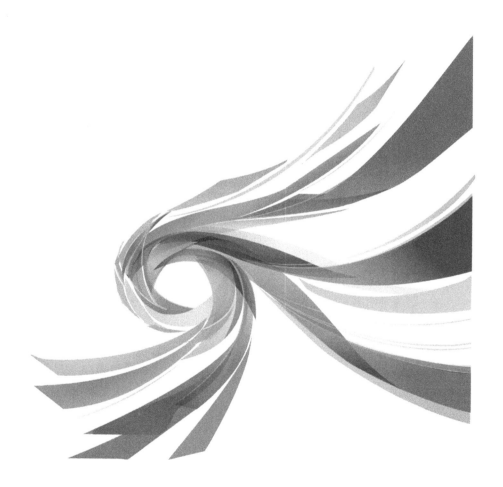

Preface by the Authors

Kelly Freeman, MSM
Founding Director, The Dysautonomia Project

Ron Crown was my dad. In 1991, at age 47, he was diagnosed with stage 4 metastatic prostate cancer. When he asked about his prognosis, he was told by his doctor, "You have time to go home and get your affairs in order." It was a death sentence. The news shocked our family. But, the way my dad responded created a ripple effect that influences my life and the lives of many today.

During the amazing nine years that followed, I watched my father become a warrior in battle—physically, emotionally, and spiritually. Because of his determination, he walked both my sister and me down the aisle and also witnessed the birth of two grandchildren.

Physically, he fought to educate himself about his condition by reading scientific-based publications and by building relationships with others who had experience with his condition. He fought to find the best doctors. He traveled out of town for consultations with experts in the field and with those who had participated in research studies. Locally, he changed doctors many times until he found a good oncologist who could be his "quarterback" for care. (He loved football!)

Emotionally, after the shock of the news hit him, he seemed to open up. He was honest and authentic as he talked about his feelings, and sometimes he would even break down and cry. But, he never allowed sorrow or pity to set in. He would allow himself time to express his feelings and then, after a few moments, he would change the subject and ask about me and how I was doing. I watched him do this with others too. He even had encounters like this with strangers, including nurses on staff at the hospitals.

Spiritually, he went through a metamorphosis. Before the cancer diagnosis, he attended church regularly. After the diagnosis, he became a passionate Christian leader. He studied the Bible daily and talked about his trust in God. He often said, "You can't become a car just by sitting in a garage. And you don't become a Christian just by sitting in church." During the last nine years of his life he counseled more people about their relationship with God than any single person I know, and in the last couple of years he had doctors referring patients to him and calling him "Dr. Crown." He was a good father and a well-respected man before he was diagnosed. He was a better man, a true role model for turning trouble into triumph, after he learned he had cancer. I wouldn't be co-authoring this book had it not been for the example he provided.

To be clear, cancer is not a good comparison to dysautonomia, which you probably already know or will learn in the coming pages. But, there are lessons to learn from his journey that apply to anyone facing a difficult health battle.

When I was initially misdiagnosed with anxiety disorder, and told to take Xanax, and to go see a counselor, I changed doctors. I was blessed to personally know a local research doctor who was willing to take on my strange case. Dr. Miguel Trevino, a contributing author and medical advisor for The Dysautonomia Project, continues to be a quarterback for my care.

Within the first few months of receiving my dysautonomia diagnosis, I started reading medical journals and participating in online discussions about the autonomic nervous system. I studied and learned as much as I could in my upright time about dysautonomia and related conditions.

My first out-of-town "medical trip" was in late 2011 to meet Dr. Randy Thompson, autonomic specialist and co-author. Randy is a doctor of autonomic medicine and also a patient. My husband and I spent 5 hours with him that first visit, a visit that gave me hope for the future of my life. I knew after that appointment that other patients needed to hear what he told us. My husband recorded and I transcribed the appointment and several since. Many of those key points are found throughout this book.

I've been a patient at many out-of-town places, and been blessed to meet several fantastic scientists of autonomic medicine in the process, many of whom are contributing authors or advisors of this book. One of those scientists is co-author Dr. David Goldstein. He is an amazing teacher who encourages me to strive for excellence and to understand concepts that once seemed far beyond my reach.

Somewhere along this journey, the enormous gap in knowledge between autonomic specialists and community-based doctors became abhorrent and unacceptable to me, and the idea for The Dysautonomia Project was born. And soon others agreed to join the project as volunteer physicians, patients, and community leaders.

The more I learn, the more I realize I don't know. I am deeply honored to join with the co-authors and contributing authors, board members, volunteers, and many others who collaborate in the development of this book, which is really a work-in-progress to transform the experience for dysautonomia patients around the world.

So, with deep gratitude for what we have and can achieve together, I invite you to join us in The Dysautonomia Project.

Kelly Freeman, MSM, a founding director of The Dysautonomia Project, is a medical writer and speaker on the topic of dysautonomias and other multi-system chronic disorders. She is also the CEO of Network People, Inc. where she has been on long term medical leave since 2011. Prior to working in information technology, she helped manage the education and training function at BayCare Health System, a large multi-hospital system in the Tampa Bay region of Florida. She has been active in her church and served as a volunteer in many community activities. In September of 2011, after sudden onset of symptoms, she was diagnosed with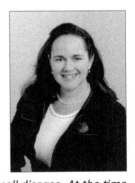
POTS, autonomically mediated syncope, and systemic mast cell disease. At the time of this publication, she is often bedridden with severe chronic orthostatic intolerance and cyclical anaphylactic/anaphylactoid circulatory shock, but lives life with a positive attitude as best she can. She is blessed by a romantic, supportive and wise husband; four children who are blossoming despite her inability to attend most of their school functions, parties and sports activities; a mother who is an encourager, friend and champion in spreading the word about dysautonomia; and an incredible number of friends, helpers, volunteers and physicians. One of her favorite things to do on Sunday mornings, when able, is to sing and play guitar with the Fillers, the praise and worship team at her church.

David S. Goldstein, MD, PhD

Clinical Neurocardiology Section
Senior Investigator, NINDS
Chief, Independent Section, CNP/DIR/NINDS
Attending Physician, NIH Clinical Center

This book is part of a growing effort to "flip the clinic" in the area of dysautonomias. For many decades the standard medical practice model in the United States has been about the same. A person feels something wrong and goes to the doctor or else goes to the doctor for a routine checkup. The doctor has the person fill out forms and questionnaires, asks questions, does a physical examination, orders tests, carries out procedures, refers to consultants, makes a diagnosis, prescribes treatments (especially medications), bills for the time and procedures, and has the person return for follow-up. My guess is that you are so used to this model you're thinking, "Well of course. What's the point? What's the alternative? And even if there were an alternative, how would it be an improvement?"

The notion of flipping the clinic draws inspiration from Sal Khan, founder of the Khan Academy. Khan Academy has sought to "flip" the classroom. Instead of listening to lectures in the classroom and doing homework at home, students listen to lectures at home and do "homework" in class, where the teacher can help students who are having difficulty and get feedback about the teaching itself. Analogously, flipping the clinic attempts to achieve two goals. The first goal is to empower patients to be more informed and engaged in their own health and health care. The second goal is to enable physicians to improve the ways they communicate with patients and support them better during and between office visits. Just as clinicians inform patients, patients inform clinicians. Each patient is like an experiment, but the "N" is 1. Support groups are also important for flipping the clinic. Not only do they relay news to patients and provide a forum for patients to compare notes and help each other, but also they can lobby effectively, provide key demographic information for scientists and policymakers, and serve as a base for recruitment into studies. In flipping the clinic, each participating group—clinicians, patients, students, caregivers, family, support groups, medical faculty—contributes to the enhancement of knowledge, which in turn informs all the groups in a kind of feedback-regulated system.

From a scientific point of view, I believe flipping the clinic will be especially valuable for patients with multi-system disorders of regulation such as dysautonomias—via a system of education, lifestyle adjustments, support groups, and internet-based outcomes research that can be compared with the standard medical practice models in terms of both cost-efficiency and patient satisfaction.

I envision an internet-based, mutually beneficial educational system that is accessible by multiple stakeholders. This book is a step in that direction because it provides a resource that both patients and clinicians can share. Through that sharing I hope the book will help flip the clinic, empowering and giving responsibility to patients with autonomic disorders.

---

*Dr. **David Goldstein** conducts patient-oriented research about autonomic and catecholamine-related disorders. He received a B.A. from Yale College in 1970 and M.D. and Ph.D. degrees from the Johns Hopkins University in 1976. He joined the National Heart, Lung, and Blood Institute in 1978, obtained tenure in 1984, and transferred to the National Institute of Neurological Disorders and Stroke in 1990. In 1999 he founded the Clinical Neurocardiology Section and has been its director ever since. An authority* 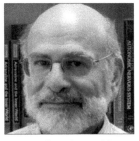 *on clinical autonomic function testing and catecholamine neurochemistry, his research has been published in 546 papers to date, including 118 first-authored, original research articles, and has been cited more than 20,000 times. Dr. Goldstein has developed numerous clinical laboratory methods, including liquid chromatography with electrochemical detection for plasma levels of catechols and 18F-dopamine scanning to visualize sympathetic innervation of the heart. His discoveries include cardiac sympathetic denervation in Parkinson's disease, differential regulation of the sympathetic noradrenergic and adrenomedullary systems in stress and distress, sympathoadrenal imbalance preceding syncope, autoimmune autonomic ganglionopathy, and a shift from vesicular uptake to oxidative deamination as a pathogenetic mechanism in Lewy-body diseases. He has received numerous awards, including two NINDS Merit Awards and the Presidential Executive Director's Award of the National Dysautonomia Research Foundation.*

Dr. Goldstein's book, Principles of Autonomic Medicine *is free and provided electronically upon email request to* www.goldsteind@ninds.nih.gov.

Charles R. Thompson, MD

Director, Center for Autonomic Disorders

When Kelly Freeman first suggested we start a website and write a book to help spread the word about dysautonomia, I just nodded my head and agreed, saying what a great thing it would be. I had heard this several times in the 15 years I have been treating this condition. And although all the ones who had wanted to do this had good intentions, the task was just too daunting, especially while suffering from this debilitating condition themselves. So while I believed her desire and would have been glad to help her, I really expected it to stop at the "want to" stage. But I didn't know Kelly. When she set her mind to do it, nothing was going to stop her, and she is the sole reason you are reading this now. And it is a story that is desperate to be told.

As a sufferer myself, I know the fatigue, dizziness, palpitations, blurred vision, chest discomfort, shortness of breath and especially the marked problems with concentration or "brain fog" that patients suffer. And the majority of the medical community know nothing of this condition or it ends up getting misdiagnosed several times before the correct diagnosis is made. The average time from symptoms to diagnosis is about 6 years. And to make it worse, this is a syndrome that affects mainly females in a 5:1 female to male ratio, usually between the ages of 12 and 45, and the majority of these are teens to early 20's.

The first diagnosis usually made is of anxiety attacks. And teenagers, no matter the sex, are just beginning to form a concept of who they are. So they begin having "attacks." Many times, the first symptom they have that brings them to medical attention is passing out. But even before that, they may have symptoms that are just blown off. This is especially true for fatigue and concentration problems. Because they look fine, they get labeled as lazy or dumb, supposedly trying to find ways of getting out of going to school. Then they pass out, all labs and x-rays and other specialized tests come back normal (ironically, what would lead to the path of diagnosis, either a tilt table test or an easy orthostatic vitals test, are not done) and the patient is labeled either "crazy" or "psycho" or some other similar tag, so then you have a young person who is so desperately trying to "fit in" or go unnoticed, becoming the butt of jokes and ridicule. And a young life that had held such promise is stigmatized, often for life.

It is not strictly teens or females who get this. For those of you who know me, you may have heard me joke that I either have an extra X chromosome or I got in touch with my feminine side. I developed this condition at age 40 and am male. I have had the loss of friends, the inability to play sports I enjoy, the inability to work full time, but the worst loss is the loss of "family time", telling your kids that something they had really been looking forward to, "I can't attend." My wife and children are saints. In 17 years, I have never seen them get upset about those types of things. But deep down, you know it has to hurt. So if this book gets some patient diagnosed quicker or helps a family member understand, then we have accomplished what we set out to do.

God bless and keep all of y'all.

Dr. Charles R. Thompson, known as "Randy" to most of his patients, received his MD from the University of Alabama, Birmingham. He is board certified in internal medi-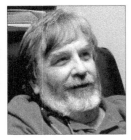cine and began his practice in 1988, in Pensacola, Florida. After a sudden onset of dysautonomia himself, he studied for one year under Cecil Coghlan of UAB, one of the founding fathers of autonomic nervous system disorders. After his fellowship with Dr. Coghlan, Randy opened the Center for Autonomic Disorders in Pensacola, Florida. Over the course of the last 15 years, he has seen more than 1500 patients with dysautonomia from more than 40 states and three other countries. These are patients desperate for answers, flying and driving to Pensacola, Florida hoping to find someone who can help. Randy is described as a "hero" by many of his patients.

CONTRIBUTORS

Lawrence B. Afrin, MD
Associate Professor of Medicine, University of Minnesota

Bonnie Black, RN, ANP
Research Coordinator, Autonomic Dysfunction Center, Vanderbilt University

Kamal R. Chemali, MD
Associate Professor of Neurology, Eastern Virginia Medical School
Director, Sentara Neuromuscular & Autonomic Center

Pradeep Chopra, MD
Assistant Professor of Medicine, Alpert Medical School, Brown University

Lisa Klimas, MS
Senior Scientist, Novartis Institute for Biomedical Research
Author & Founder, *MastAttack.org*

Alan Pocinki, MD, FACP
Clinical Associate Professor of Medicine, George Washington University

David Robertson, MD
Professor of Medicine & Pharmacology and Neurology
Elton Yates Professor of Autonomic Disorders
Director, Autonomic Research Center, Vanderbilt University Autonomic

Julian Stewart, MD, PhD
Professor of Pediatrics, Physiology & Medicine
Director, Center for Hypotension, New York Medical College

Miguel Trevino, MD
Medical Director, Innovative Research Center
Director, Center for Hypotension, New York Medical College

Steven Vernino, MD, PhD
Professor & Academic Vice Chair,
Department of Neurology & Neurotherapeutics
University of Texas Southwestern Medical Center

MEDICAL ADVISORS

Daniel Cabello, MD
Neurologist and Epileptologist,
Clinical Neurosciences of Tampa Bay, Clearwater, FL
The Dysautonomia Project Local Medical Advisory Board & CME Speaker

Glen Cook, MD
Neurophysiology & Autonomic Disorders Specialist,
Department of Neurology
Naval Medical Center Portsmouth, VA

Paul Phillips, MD, FACC
Cardiologist, Clearwater Cardiovascular Consultants, Clearwater, FL
The Dysautonomia Project Local Medical Advisory Board

Satish Raj, MD, MSCI, FACC
Associate Professor of Cardiac Services
Libin Cardiovascular Institute of Alberta, Canada

Doug Welpton, MD
Psychiatrist, Author & Speaker
The Dysautonomia Project Board of Directors
and Local Medical Advisory Board

SUPPORTING AUTHOR

Kaylee Sills
Chapters 30 & 32
4th Year Nursing Student at Indiana Wesleyan University,
Assistant Director, Dysautonomia Advocacy Foundation

SPECIAL CONTRIBUTIONS

A special thanks goes out to Karen Crown, President and founder of The Dysautonomia Project. Without her passion about the need for education in the local community to help other patients, like her daughter, this organization and book would not have been created.

To Nate Freeman, founding board member and supportive husband, without whose continuous encouragement this book would have remained "a good idea."

Thank you to the amazing leadership team that surpassed all expectations in the first year as a new not-for-profit organization—the inaugural Board of Directors for The Dysautonomia Project, including Polly Stannard, Ali Key, Kirk Blank, Melinda Ferm, Andrea Layman, Beth Pike, Molly duPont Schaffer, Dr. Doug Welpton, and Mary Elizabeth Welpton.

Thank you to all our local medical advisors, including Dr. Daniel Cabello, Dr. Ernesto Meyer, Dr. Laura Meyer, Dr. Ron Perrott, Dr. Paul Phillips, Dr. Miguel Trevino, and Dr. Doug Welpton, who have all helped to shape the project by walking with us in learning about dysautonomia and applying lessons learned in their practices.

Thank you to all the Dysautonomia Project volunteers, without whom we would not be successful. A few that have helped shape this book through feedback and personal examples are Myrna Concepcion, Heather McEvilly, Lisa Rooker, Ainsley Glenn, Laurie LaLacheur, Nancy Bennett, Dianne Freeman, Maranda Parr, Nicolette Hamp, Amy Kleinlein, Jenna Yates, Tara Johnson, Julie Swink, Deniz McClure, Donna Huebsch, Jim Kendall, Amanda Jackson, Laura Pearson, Michelle Wolford, Susan Smith, Tava Wilson, Tony Degina, and Ashleigh Pike.

This book would not be possible without the preceding effort of many other not-for-profit organizations and leaders of online discussions, apps and facebook pages. Many have influenced this book but a few that have been instrumental in inspiring the pages that follow include Dysautonomia Information Network (DINET.org) and its private online forum; Dysautonomia Advocacy Foundation and its prolific facebook page; Dysautonomia Youth Network of America; POTSUK.org; Kim, of POTSY PRAISE, Laurie, of The Faces of Dysatuonomia; Jill and Mike, of the Stand App and the Potsies Count online survey, the creative team at Symple (a mobile health tracking app), Lisa, of Florida Teens & Parents of POTS facebook page and Lisa, of *Mastattack.org*.

Thank you to Deborah J. Cornwall, who introduced our organization to publisher Chris Angermann of Bardolf & Company. Chris has been a perfect fit in helping to put the pieces of this book together. He has been patient, exacting, funny and ferociously honest at just the right times. Thank you Cathleen Shaw for a beautiful cover design. And thanks to Leatrice Malak for her copy editing.

And finally, thank you to Elizabeth Freeman, creator of our organizational logo, for a brilliant design that sums up without words what most patients with dysautonomia feel each time they stand upright.

HOW TO USE THIS BOOK FOR PATIENTS

The goal of this book is to provide a starting point for patients, family members, and others who want to understand the basic nature of dys-autonomia and learn how to live with this con-dition. You'll notice that most even-numbered pages are aimed at the patient, and that the ma-terial corresponds to the information for phy-sicians found on the opposite (odd-numbered) pages.

> *Most of the even-numbered pages are written for the patient.*

Some chapters are written by subject experts, and their names appear on the initial page along with this logo. Most of the rest are a collaborative effort by the co-au-thors, Kelly Freeman, David S. Goldstein, and Charles R. Thompson. Chapters 30 and 32 also benefited from the research and medical writing of Kaylee Sills.

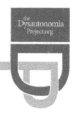

In this book you will learn:

- How the autonomic nervous system (ANS) is designed to func-tion properly;

- What may happen when the ANS doesn't work properly = dysautonomia(s);

- The difference between autonomic dysfunction and auto-nomic failure;

- What to expect in working with doctor(s), and tips that can help;

- What you need to know about getting a correct diagnosis;

- If diagnosed, what you can expect in the short-term and long-term;

- Lots of information about various kinds of treatments, found both in the book and at *www.TheDysautono-miaProject.org*;

How to Use This book for Physicians

This book is a starting point for physicians, patients, and others to understand the basic etiology and pathophysiology of autonomic nervous system (ANS) disorders. It is also a functional reference tool in the clinic for physicians who are not specialists in dysautonomia. Most even-numbered pages are for patients, while corresponding medical information for physicians appears on the opposite (odd-numbered) pages.

> *Most corresponding odd-numbered pages are written for the physician.*

Some chapters are written by subject experts, and their names appear on the initial page along with this logo. Most of the rest are a collaborative effort by the co-authors, Kelly Freeman, David S. Goldstein, MD, PhD, and Charles R. Thompson, MD. Chapters 30 and 32 also benefited from the research and medical writing of Kaylee Sills.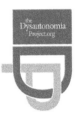

The book provides information so that physicians can provide:

- A thorough, initial clinical assessment;
- Important patient education upon diagnosis;
- Referrals to appropriate local specialists and/or major medical centers for further autonomic function testing;
- Proper interpretations and understanding of the results of the most common autonomic tests;
- Treatment and follow-ups for dysautonomia patients as needed.

Ideally, physicians would review this book in its entirety after completing "The Dysautonomia Project Grand Rounds CME Course." Additionally, this book serves as a reference guide and educational tool for the physician, other health care practitioners, and patients in the clinic or hospital setting.

- Many tips and ideas that may be helpful for learning to live with dysautonomia.

First, it is important to understand what dysautonomia is so that you can make wise decisions about treatment options.

A NOTE FOR FAMILY MEMBERS

We recognize that family members of patients will be reading this book; however, we've purposefully directed the writing of these pages to the patient because:

- Dysautonomia can affect people of varying ages.
- To the extent that it's appropriate, it helps younger patients to take charge of their own care.

That said, we do believe that family members will find these pages a useful guide for talking about the medical condition.

On the website *www.TheDysautonomiaProject.org* you will find a fantastic set of resources, including several suggestions for tools and aids that may help you as you live with dysautonomia. You'll also see links to many outstanding articles, videos, and reputable websites where you can discover great additional information and even connect with other patients.

By using this book and sharing its contents, together we build hope for the future.

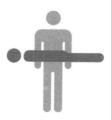

Most odd-numbered pages are written for both primary care and specialty care physicians, nurse practitioners, and medical students. The pages are designed to provide both clinically relevant data with supporting references to validated research, as well as findings from in-clinic observations and follow-ups of dysautonomia patients during the past 15 years. The aim is to provide high-level information for the busy physician who does not have time to become an expert in this area of study. (Even numbered pages, designed for the patient, summarize the same topic in lay terms and often add additional information, including helpful tips, diagrams, and tools that may aid the patient living with dysautonomia.)

On The Dysautonomia Project website you will find resources for greater clinical understanding. Available are several outstanding, evidence-based publications, including "Primer of the Autonomic Nervous System" compiled by David Robertson et al., "Adrenaline and the Inner World: An Introduction to Scientific Integrative Medicine" by David S. Goldstein, MD, PhD, and other exceptional publications from contributing authors and other experts in the dysautonomia field. Additional helpful resources include links to relevant clinical research and websites. Visit *www.TheDysautonomiaProject.org* to download free resources and tools such as the "Orthostatic Vitals Test" and "Clinical Assessment Forms" for evaluating dysautonomias.

This book is also available for purchase in an eBook format.

To help users, the 5 main points are summarized in Section 1: "Five Things to Know."

By using this book, sharing its contents, and collaborating with the authors by giving feedback for continuous improvement, together we will build hope for the future.

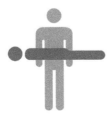

FOREWORD

DAVID ROBERTSON, MD

In *The Dysautonomia Project,* Kelly Freeman, David Goldstein and Charles Thompson have created a wonderful resource that reflects the spectrum of the broad aspect of dysautonomia. What is different about this book is the collaboration of patients with dysautonomia, physicians expert in dysautonomias, and community leaders and, indeed, the general public. Of greatest importance are the patients and family members who have suffered, in many cases, for their loved one to get a proper diagnosis. This book tries and succeeds to mesh these different perspectives into an excellent, readable and inspirational labor of love that is dedicated to all those and their loved ones who have frequently, in the past, found it difficult to identify an easily accessible level of information. In the case of postural tachycardia syndrome, many relatively young patients may have this disorder for many years and, characteristically often, receive no specific diagnosis because postural tachycardia syndrome has diverse causes and those causes may be quite different in different individuals.

In situations like this the frustration of patients can be unrelenting, and they may be unable to get a diagnosis or may even be told that perhaps they don't really have a disease. Thankfully, as the information about autonomic disorders has permeated the news media more recently, patients are learning to identify new sources of information.

The most important aspect of *The Dysautonomia Project* is that the authors have pulled together all of the problems from a human standpoint for people who are affected by dysautonomia. They have gone further by not only describing places where patients and family members can learn about dysautonomia, but also by encouraging patients, and their families, to understand that obtaining this knowledge is absolutely critical.

Some autonomic diseases are extremely debilitating and, in many cases, that is very obvious to friends, relatives, and neighbors. In other cases, different dysautonomias may take a very great toll on the patient's life and yet the patient may look as healthy as anyone else. In many cases the problems of dysautonomia lie inside the patient in ways that are not easily seen, and the "invisible illness" is yet another burden with which the patient must live.

With this new book, accessible through the Internet and in print, life may well be better for the patients with the illness and their family members who have not had full access to the sources of information and guidance of physicians experienced in the care of dysautonomia patients.

There is another aspect to this book that will be of fundamental importance to those of us who care for these patients. There is a plea that all of us physicians should take the time to provide the appropriate care and to be supportive in how we interact with our patients. The authors identify Cecil Coghlan, MD, in Birmingham, Alabama for the enormous number of patients with dysautonomias that he cared for over his very long life. Most of us recognized that Cecil was totally dedicated to the support of his patients. Those of us who knew Cecil will feel that the book's dedication is entirely appropriate.

David Robertson, MD is Professor of Neurology & Director, Autonomic Dysfunction Research Center, Vanderbilt University, Nashville, TN. Dr. Robertson received his medical degree from Vanderbilt University Medical School in 1973. He went on to complete an internship and residency in Medicine at Johns Hopkins Hospital. Robertson was a postdoctoral fellow in Clinical Pharmacology at Vanderbilt for two years before accepting a position as assistant chief of Service in Medicine and instructor in Medicine at Johns Hopkins in 1977. Along with his current roles as professor of Medicine and Pharmacology and professor of Neurology, 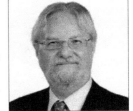 *Robertson is currently the Elton Yates Professor of Autonomic Disorders, director of the General Clinical Research Center and director of the Center for Space Physiology and Medicine for Vanderbilt University.*

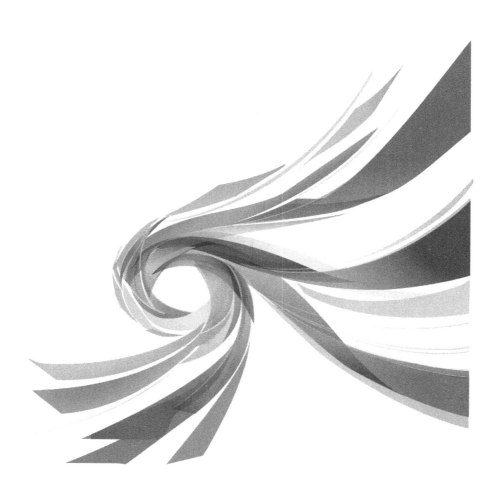

SECTION 1

FIVE THINGS TO KNOW

IF YOU READ NOTHING ELSE, READ THIS

Before we begin, I will tell you, "Nothing you say about your symptoms will surprise me."

Dr. Randy Thompson's first words to Kelly and Nate Freeman during their initial appointment at the Center for Autonomic Dysfunction

I

BATTLE #I

MOST PATIENTS ARE MISDIAGNOSED

Dysautonomia may be one of the most often overlooked and misdi-agnosed conditions of all time, making the goal of getting a correct diagnosis the first battle for the patient and family. Unless you happen upon a well-trained doctor, the battle requires:

- Unrelenting determination to get an accurate diagnosis;
- Documenting symptoms and having open discussions with your doctor(s) to share specific facts about your symptoms, including the onset of the symptoms;
- A willingness to change your doctor if he or she does not seek to fully understand your case and work with you to find answers.

Here are a few facts relevant to this often misdiagnosed condition:

- Dysautonomia is not a disease or diagnosis. It is a general term used to describe a disor-der of the autonomic nervous system (ANS).

- The ANS is more commonly known as the automatic nervous system because it con-trols the bodily functions that we don't consciously control, such as blood pressure, digestion, and perspiration.

- Dysautonomias have a specific set of symp-toms involving malfunctions or failure of the ANS. (See "The Dysautonomia Universe," Chapter 8.)

> *Dysautonomias have a specific set of symptoms involving malfunctions or failure of the autonomic nervous system.*

- The average time to a diagnosis is currently 6 years.[1]
- 83% of patients are inappropriately diagnosed with anxiety dis-order or other psychological disorders before they are diagnosed appropriately.[2]

I

BATTLE #I

MOST PATIENTS ARE MISDIAGNOSED

For the physician untrained in treating patients with autonomic nervous system (ANS) dysfunction or failure, diagnosis is a battle confounded by the difficulty in balancing "do no harm" with the ever increasing organizational pressures to see more patients in less time. In clinic, the average American primary care physician aims to spend less than 15 minutes with the follow-up patient.[1] Yet, the undiagnosed patient with dysautonomia has a large array of multi-organ problems that are widely heterogeneous. One patient's main complaint may be nausea, while the next patient's primary complaint is migraine headaches. The patient complaints are often so numerous and varied that, in most cases, patients focus on their biggest concern and fail to report the full extent of their symptoms. Thus, it is up to the physician to elucidate the full extent of the symptom load.

Case Example: The patient being examined is anxious to understand what is wrong. She hasn't been feeling like herself and begins to describe her problems. As the patient speaks about her symptoms, her norepinephrine levels surge, her heart rate elevates, and mild bronchial constriction makes her breathing slightly labored. Since the patient is a woman of childbearing age who has complaints of palpitations and irregularity in sweating, the untrained physician explains that these complaints are common for anxiety disorder. A script for low dose Xanax is written, and the patient is given a list of counselors in the local area.

Meanwhile, lurking underneath the easier-to-assess integumentary, orthopedic, pulmonary, digestive, and cardiac systems of this patient

- Few doctors learn about dysautonomia in medical school. In early March 2014, Ken Kaufman, MD, Chief Resident for OB/GYN at Bayfront Medical Center in St. Petersburg, Florida, stated that he only had "one short lecture" in medical school that touched on autonomic dysfunction. He recalled, "It had something to do with spinal cord injuries." It is unclear if the lecture included the term "dysautonomia."

[1,2] Deborah J. Cornwall, "Invisible Illness: How to Sustain Hope," *Huffington Post*, July 11, 2014. (Data reported from a survey of more than 400 dysautonomia patients conducted by Dysautonomia International in 2014.)

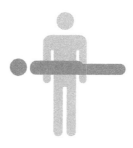

are a number of difficult-to-assess, microscopic breakdowns that are creating abnormal norepinephrine (NE) levels in the sympathetic nerves, which are causing dysfunction[2] of the ANS, and thereby are creating a physiological inability to maintain homeostasis. Yet, most lab tests are within normal limits.

This common scenario illustrates how misdiagnosis of this invisible illness is so pervasive. Eighty-three percent of patients are misdiagnosed with a psychiatric condition prior to a more accurate diagnosis involving ANS disorders.[3] While the pressure on physicians to assess and diagnose quickly is problematic, the greater issue is that most physicians have not been properly trained about dysautonomia. And that is the aim of this book—to provide physicians with the basic knowledge and an easy-to-use set of tools needed to speed the time to an accurate diagnosis.

> *Anxiety disorder is a diagnosis of exclusion...the patient has no background at this moment to suggest generalized anxiety disorder... For that reason I insist on trying to rule out other possible explanations, such as pheocromcytoma, Guillian-Barré syndrome, atypical migraines, dysautonomia, or other conditions that may present with a clinical picture similar to panic attacks.*

Daniel Cabello, MD
Consulting Neurologist
September 28, 2011

---

[1] Miguel Trevino, quote regarding challenges facing community-based physicians treating patients with dysautonomia. Largo, Florida, 2014.

[2] NE is one of the main chemical messengers of the ANS. It is the main chemical messenger of the sympathetic noradrenergic nervous system. When not regulated properly, it is known to create dysfunction of the ANS.

[3] Deborah J. Cornwall, "Invisible Illness: How to Sustain Hope," *Huffington Post*, July 11, 2014. (Data reported from a survey of more than 400 dysautonomia patients conducted by Dysautonomia International in 2014.)

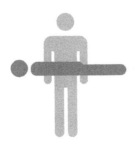

2

EASY TO ASSESS

With The Right Knowledge

by Kelly Freeman

My hairstylist's name is Melinda. She has done my hair for years, and after my illness she witnessed an enormous change in me. Before I got sick, I was perhaps one of her most active, outgoing, busy working mom clients. After the onset of my condition, I barely had the strength to open the door and walk into the salon. I wore sunglasses and earplugs because of the bright lights and sounds. I had to prop my feet up and get up very slowly to prevent feelings of lightheadedness and fainting. Melinda asked lots of questions about what had happened and, over the following months, witnessed my ups and downs in energy level, functioning, and mental alertness.

> *How can it be that my hairstylist can recognize dysautonomia when an overwhelming majority of local physicians overlook it?*

About a year after I became disabled, Melinda called to tell me she had another client who was experiencing similar symptoms to mine. She asked if that client could call me to talk about what was happening to us. We did meet, and soon afterwards Melinda's client was diagnosed with POTS, the same form of dysautonomia I have. Since then Melinda has referred three other clients to me, all either diagnosed with a form of dysautonomia or suspicious for dysautonomia.

How can it be that my hairstylist can recognize dysautonomia when an overwhelming majority of local physicians overlook it? Or misdiagnose it?

She gained the right knowledge.

2

EASY TO ASSESS

WITH KNOWLEDGE OF KEY SIGNS AND SYMPTOMS

There is very little in physician education on autonomic disorders.

Thomas Chelimsky, MD
Past President,
American Autonomic Society

In about 15 minutes in the clinic, you can get a fairly good idea if there is something going on with the autonomic nervous system, if you ask thoughtful questions about the patient's history, including questions about common signs and symptoms of dysautonomia. If you suspect dysautonomia is involved, both a comprehensive clinical assessment and an Orthostatic Vitals Test may be warranted. (See Section III for details about assessing the dysautonomia patient.)

If, while taking the patient's case history, you notice a pattern of complaints that fit with several of the common symptom categories: fatigue, pre-syncope/syncope, neurological and/or gastrointestinal complaints, orthostatic intolerance/hypotension and/or pulmonary difficulties— then you have uncovered clues that dysautonomia might be present and needs to be ruled out. Once dysautonomia is suspected it is important to follow with a comprehensive clinical assessment.

A nurse or other trained office staff can conduct an orthostatic vitals test in the clinic. Alternatively, you can schedule a tilt table test. After a comprehensive clinical assessment (which takes longer than 15 minutes if done properly) and an orthostatic vitals test, you will have enough meaningful information about the patient's current medical history, including measurable variables with reported symptoms

Over the course of studying and learning more about my own condition, I would share my knowledge with her during our appointments. She witnessed the signs and symptoms of my condition over a long period of time. When seeing other clients and talking with them about their symptoms, she began to connect the dots. Although she had not read a single medical journal on the topic, she knew the top clues that suggest it might be dysautonomia. These clues are discussed in Chapter 10. This is a great chapter to read if you suspect that you, or someone you know, might have dysautonomia.

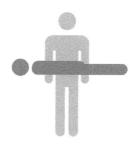

while experiencing orthostatic stress, to support an initial proper diagnosis.

While at first glance the clinically measurable hemodynamic variations appear to be the most relevant factor in assessing dysautonomia, the trained physician knows that the most important data is the information collected while talking with the patient.

Top 7 Signs and Symptoms of Dysautonomia

1. Difficulty Standing Still
2. Fatigue
3. Lightheadedness
4. Nausea and Other GI Symptoms
5. Brain Fog or Mental Clouding
6. Palpitations or Chest Discomfort
7. Shortness of Breath or Difficulty Breathing

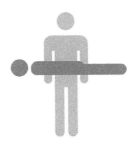

3

A MEANINGFUL DIAGNOSIS

A BETTER CHANCE
AT GETTING BETTER

If you've been told you have dysautono-mia, that's a good start. But if you have a chronic debilitating condition involving dysautonomia, it is not a good stopping point. To understand if you should pursue further diagnostic testing for a more mean-ingful diagnosis, ask yourself this question:

> *Dysautonomia is not a diagnosis. It is a term used to describe any disorder of the autonomic (automatic) nervous system.*

Do I go places and do things like other people?

If you answered "yes," then pursuing further diagnostic testing may be unnecessary, as you likely have an episodic or mild case. Working with local physicians to find the right treatment plan aimed at improving and preventing symptoms is sufficient.

If your answer is "no," then digging deeper to better understand the mechanisms and/or coexisting conditions that either cause or exacer-bate symptoms will help you and your physician pursue treatment op-tions better targeted at your more complex case. It is important to note that it is not always possible to find the underlying cause.

Dysautonomia is not a diagnosis. It is a term used to describe any disor-der of the autonomic (automatic) nervous system. A meaningful diagno-sis includes:

- Identifying what form of dysautonomia you have (for more see Chapters 8 and 9);

- Knowing what co-existing conditions you have (such as sleep apnea, gastroparesis, etc.);

3

A MEANINGFUL DIAGNOSIS

IMPROVING PATIENT OUTCOMES

If the assessment process reveals both abnormal hemodynamic signs through orthostatic testing, and a pattern of symptoms consistent with abnormal functioning of the ANS, as revealed through the clinical assessment, including a detailed patient case history, it is then important to identify an accurate dysautonomia diagnosis. Initially this involves determining a definitive dysautonomia diagnosis. (See Chapters 8, "The "Dysautonomia Universe" and 9, "Orthostatic Intolerance Spectrum," for more about specific dysautonomia classifications.)

When a patient presents with a transient form of orthostatic intolerance, and/or symptoms of chronic orthostatic intolerance that are mild in nature, it is often sufficient to hold off on further testing and begin trialing non-pharmacological approaches to treatment. In some cases of mild but chronic orthostatic intolerance, it may be helpful to consider whether the patient is a candidate for first line pharmacological treatments as well. The assessment serves as a baseline test and is a good measure for following the patient over time. In many cases, patients with transient or mild forms of dysautonomia are able to carry out their daily activities with mild adaptation and a tolerable treatment regime.

Achieving a more meaningful diagnosis is important when a patient's case appears more complex and/or the patient is experiencing disabling symptoms that interfere with the normal activities of daily living. In these cases, it is important to consider other tests for dysautonomia, including physiological tests, neuropharmacological tests, and, in some cases, genetic tests. (See chapter 17 for more about autonomic function testing.) Just as there is not one single form of dysautonomia, there is

- Understanding what is causing the dysautonomia. Is it the primary condition?

Those who are successful in identifying the primary cause are often the most successful in improving their overall health. However, for most patients, getting at the deeper root cause of dysautonomia takes time, persistence, and further diagnostic testing. Some patients, even after years, don't find the definitive underlying cause; but, in the process of trying, they often learn how to better deal with their condition.

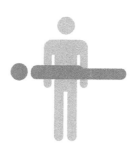

not one single test, beyond that of the initial clinical assessment, indicated for all dysautonomia patients. In patients with debilitating chronic orthostatic intolerance or forms of adult onset autonomic failure, seek to identify the primary condition that creates and/or exacerbates the ANS disorder. In cases where the primary condition is effectively treated, the dysautonomia symptoms usually improve. It may be helpful to identify where the patient falls in the Dysautonomia Universe and/or on the Orthostatic Intolerance Spectrum found in chapters 8 and 9. In these cases, digging deeper to gain clues about known mechanisms that contribute to ANS difficulties can sometimes be discovered by further diagnostic testing. Such clinical evidence will result in a more meaningful diagnosis and, ultimately, a better treatment plan.

Understanding various known mechanisms involved in ANS disorders, such as catecholamine abnormalities, hypovolemia, venous pooling, vascular permeability, small fiber neuropathies, mast cell activation disorders, and other coexisting conditions (discussed in other chapters), may be especially helpful in selecting the most effective treatment options. For instance, a patient who is pooling a lot of blood upon orthostasis (which may be evidenced by a narrowing pulse pressure on standing[1] and visual signs of cyanosis or edema in the feet), may respond better to pharmacological treatments that are known vasoconstrictors than to drugs that will help increase plasma volume.

---

[1] Streeten, DH et al. "Abnormal Orthostatic Changes in blood pressure and heart rate in subjects with intact sympathetic nervous function: evidence for excessive venous pooling." J Lab Clin Med. 1988 Mar; 111 (3): 326-35.

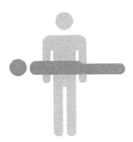

4

BATTLE #2

TREATMENT REQUIRES
PATIENCE AND PERSEVERANCE

Once diagnosed with a form of dysautonomia, the bigger, more daunting battle begins: finding the right treatment(s.)

Why? Unlike a diagnosis of appendicitis, in which patients tend to have consistent symptoms of a limited spectrum, patients with forms of dysautonomia can experience a wide assortment of problems. Therefore, a wide assortment of treatments must be tested and tried with the aim of improving the overall health and ability of the patient to function.

	Appendicitis	Rich, a patient with POTS, a chronic form of dysautonomia
Problem(s)	Pain in the lower right abdomen	Abdominal pain, overwhelming fatigue, headaches, nausea, insomnia, lightheadedness, occasional fainting, difficulty breathing, chest pain, palpitations, constipation, diarrhea, pins and needles tingling in his hands and feet, excessive sweating, heat intolerance and brain fog.
Assessment	Physical Exam, CT Scan	Clinical Assessment, orthostatic vitals
Treatment	Surgical Removal of Appendix	**Currently:** high salt diet, high fluid intake, mild exercise, pyridostigmine, clonazepam, and amphetamines. **Previously tried and discontinued:** SNRI, fludrocortisone, beta-blockers, clonidine, sumatriptan, midodrine, compression stockings.
Recovery	Approximately 5-10 days	unknown
Patient	Can rely on the doctor to assess, treat and follow-up to ensure there are no complications.	Must try different treatment approaches, one at a time, noting changes in symptoms and side effects, and working with his doctor to find the best treatment combination.

Each patient with Postural Orthostatic Tachycardia Syndrome (POTS) is different. This is one example. Other patients with POTS may have different problems, diagnostic tests, and treatments.

4

BATTLE #2

TREATMENT REQUIRES
PATIENCE AND PERSEVERANCE

Since there is no known cause for primary, or idiopathic, dysautonomia, treatment is generally aimed at symptom management. If the dysautonomia is secondary to a known primary condition, a combined approach should be used:

- Improve the primary condition.
- Manage dysautonomia symptoms.

The more complex the case, the greater the need for patience and persistence in trialing various treatment options to find the most helpful combination.

Both pharmacological and non-pharmacological interventions should be considered when developing the treatment plan. Pharmacological treatments may include volume expanders, beta-blockers, benzodiazepines, vasoconstrictors, among a long list of others. The need for non-pharmacological treatments cannot be overstated and, in some cases, may be sufficient in providing effective symptom improvement. Such treatments may include exercise, a high salt diet, compression garments, and increasing fluid intake, among others. (See section V for both summary and comprehensive lists of generally accepted pharmacological and non-pharmacological treatments.)

Due to the heterogeneous presentation of dysautonomia patients, treatment plans must be individualized. Treatments that are effective with some patients may exacerbate symptoms in other patients.

Before embarking on a treatment plan, consider any known coexisting conditions. This is important, as many patients with more complex conditions may experience adverse reactions to certain drug classes

The Top Two Things To Do

1. Study and learn all you can about dysautonomia. (Even if the thought is overwhelming, try to learn one new thing each week. This book is a great start.)

2. Become your own patient advocate by keeping a journal of symptoms that correspond with your changes in treatment.

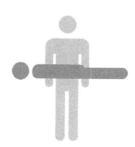

and even non-pharmacological measures. For instance, patients with coexisting systemic mast cell disease are known to respond poorly to beta-blockers which can cause mast cell degranulation. Patients with known intermittent gastroparesis respond poorly to a diet high in cellulose fiber due to the low motility of the GI tract.

When educating patients about their treatment plan, it is crucial to emphasize the importance of changing only one variable at a time. Encourage patients to keep a journal or record of their symptoms to track trends in improvement and/or side effects noticed as each treatment changes.

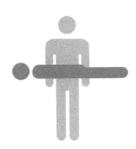

5

IMPORTANT EXPECTATIONS
THREE GOALS, FIVE TIPS
AND ONE MYTH

This is a marathon, not a sprint.
Dr. Randy Thompson

Three Goals

1. To have more good days and fewer bad days;
2. To use tools to help improve your ability to lead as normal and independent a life as possible;
3. To find meaning, purpose and joy in the new normal.

Five Tips

1. Be flexible. Make plans with the knowledge that they may change at the last minute.
2. When the fatigue and/or pain sets in, give in to it. Don't try to fight it.
3. Exercise as best you can to strengthen both the large skeletal muscles of your body and the small smooth muscles of your vascular system. Any kind of movement is good.
4. Graze or eat several small meals during the day. Avoid big and/or high starch meals to keep blood from pooling in the many blood vessels that surround your digestive system.
5. Shop efficiently. Know what you need, walk into a store quickly, get what you need, and get out. Avoid busy shopping times with long lines where you have to stand and wait.

5

IMPORTANT EXPECTATIONS
When Following Patients

Dysautonomias are Mind-Body Disorders that Require a Systems Approach

Possibly more than any other condition, dysautonomia is a set of mind-body disorders. This can be a difficult concept for both patients and physicians because traditionally we treat mind disorders by sending patients to psychiatrists or psychologists; and, we treat body disorders initially in the primary or acute care setting, and then by the specialist or subspecialist who has an expertise about a specific region of the body. The autonomic nervous system (ANS), however, operates at the very border of both the mind and the body and involves multiple organ systems. The ANS is responsible for the internal adjustments that accompany every motion a person performs and every emotion a person feels. Because of this interconnected association, it is important to:

- Consider a "systems approach" in treating the patient. What might be an ideal treatment for constipation for most patients, (e.g. eating a diet high in fiber) may not be the ideal treatment for the patient with dysautonomia because this treatment may cause too much blood to pool in the splanchnic bed and shunt an abnormal supply of blood away from vital organs.

- Avoid assessing symptoms at first glance. What appears at first glance to be anxiety due to an emotional reaction may actually be abnormal chemical release mediated by an internal physiological abnormality such as a catecholamine disorder (e.g. what looks like a panic attack may be an abnormal

One Myth: Most Patients Faint
The Truth: Most Patients Don't Faint

The clinical term for fainting is syncope (syn-co-pee). While dysautonomia symptoms are often made worse by an upright posture, only about 40% of people with dysautonomia actually pass out.[1] In those cases, it may be only once or twice. About 85% of POTS patients present with the triad of dizziness/lightheadedness, nausea, and debilitating fatigue.[2]

If you hear someone say, "You can't have dysautonomia because you've never passed out." You can tell them, "Fainting is not a requirement for dysautonomia. That's just a myth."

---

[1] Thompson, Charles R. Interview. Pensacola, Florida; December, 2011.

[2] Deborah J. Cornwall, "Invisible Illness: How to Sustain Hope," *Huffington Post*, July 11, 2014

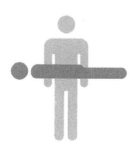

release of adrenaline causing palpitations, dilation of blood vessels in the large muscles, hyperventilation and/or bronchial constriction).

- Pain and stress are the top two enemies of dysautonomia. Why? Because pain and stress trigger the fight-or-flight response to a given situation, which may cause the release of chemical mediators such as catecholamines, neurotransmitters, hormones and/or cytokines that can potentially over stimulate the sympathetic nervous system. When this occurs, it is as if the system goes into overdrive, like revving the engine of a car in the garage. Or the reverse could happen, a marked drop in norepinephrine could cause an abnormal parasympathetic response, like the car stalling out due to lack of appropriate fuel. (See more about the top enemies of dysautonomia in Chapter 26.)

- Dysautonomia affects family and friends. Patients with dysautonomia often don't "look sick," which is why some, including parents and/or spouses, have a hard time believing the condition is "real." Although it may, at times, appear that the patient is just being lazy, in reality, many patients are trapped in bodies that are trying unsuccessfully to maintain homeostasis. This invisible illness has the potential to cause significant conflict with friends and family members who do not understand dysautonomia (e.g. The family has plans to go to a party, but the patient who felt fine enough to attend might suddenly be overcome with fatigue, nausea, and/or pain and have to cancel at the last minute. The plans for the family then must change). Therefore it is important that family members and friends are educated about dysautonomia.

- Managing time in the clinic can be difficult. Since patients have a wide assortment of complaints, and varying levels of understanding, they undoubtedly require more extended interactions than the average follow-up patient. Determining how to manage time before entering the exam room is helpful. Some physicians schedule appointments with dysautonomia patients at the end of the morning or end of the day.

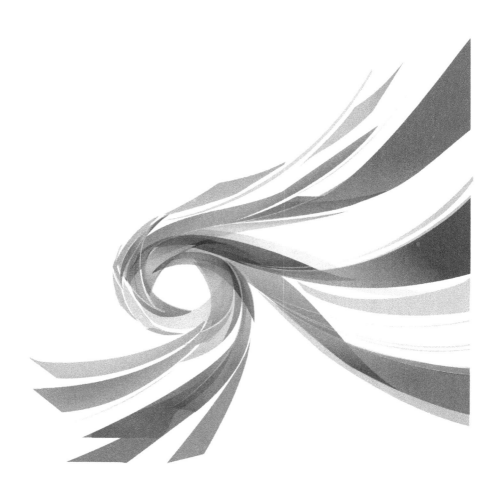

SECTION 2

ABOUT DYSAUTONOMIAS

WHEN THE INNER WORLD OF THE BODY DOESN'T WORK RIGHT

Our bodies are made of extraordinarily unstable material. Pulses of energy, so minute that very delicate methods are required to measure them, course along our nerves. On reaching muscles they find there a substance so delicately sensitive to slight disturbance that, like an explosive touched off by a fuse, it may discharge in a powerful movement.

Walter B. Cannon
Introducing the concept of Homeostasis
Wisdom of the Body, 1932

6

HOW THE AUTONOMIC NERVOUS SYSTEM WORKS

HOMEOSTASIS IS THE AIM

I think my body has forgotten about 98.6°F.

Kelly Freeman, July 5, 2015
Outside Lambeau Field in Green Bay, Wisconsin.
View video at
www.TheDysautonomiaProject.org/Resources/1

The nervous system of the body is by far the least understood of all body systems. It is made up of an overwhelmingly complex network of neurons electrically charged and dynamically changed by a vast number of chemical messengers produced in places all over the body.

The nervous system of the body can be divided two ways. By structure, it is identified by its location in the body as either the central or peripheral nervous system. By function, the somatic or autonomic nervous systems control different parts of the body.

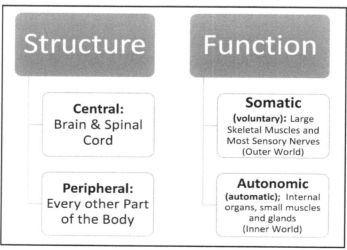

Structure	Function
Central: Brain & Spinal Cord	**Somatic** (**voluntary**): Large Skeletal Muscles and Most Sensory Nerves (Outer World)
Peripheral: Every other Part of the Body	**Autonomic** (**automatic**); Internal organs, small muscles and glands (Inner World)

6

HOW THE AUTONOMIC NERVOUS SYSTEM WORKS

STRUCTURE AND FUNCTION

The coordinated physiological processes which maintain most of the steady states in the organism are so complex and so peculiar to living beings—involving, as they may, the brain and nerves, the heart, lungs, kidneys and spleen, all working cooperatively—that I have suggested a special designation for these states, homeostasis.

Walter B. Cannon, 1932

Homeostasis, the aim of the autonomic nervous system, depends on a wide array of variables that affect the body to be intact and to function properly. These variables can be divided into three general categories: structure, function, and chemical messengers.

Structure

The structure of the central nervous system includes the brain and the spinal cord. The spinal cord can be divided into three sections: cervical, thoracolumbar, and sacral.

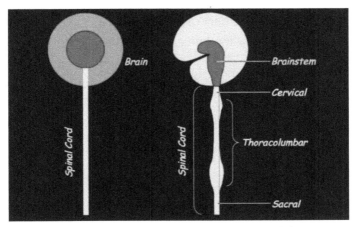

The central nervous system is like a tootsie roll pop divided into sections.

Of these divisions, the autonomic nervous system receives little attention in medical education today. Yet, the autonomic nervous system
(ANS) plays a role in essentially every aspect of the life of the body. Its
aim is to achieve homeostasis, a steady state of the inner world of the
body, and it does this by enabling the body to adapt to variables such
as temperature and gravity.

The ANS operates much like an air conditioner
in a house. An air conditioner has a thermostat that helps regulate proper temperature
in all the rooms. Many variables may affect
a room's temperature, including the season
of the year, as well as the number of people,
the placement of vents, and the amount of
lighting in the room. If the room is uncomfort-
ably cool, we can go to the thermostat and
turn its air temperature up. If the system is

> *The ANS uses
> many internal au-
> tomatic regulators,
> like thermostats,
> to maintain
> a fairly steady
> state in the inner
> world of our body.*

working properly, in a relatively short period of time the room will
become more comfortable. The air conditioner's thermostat helps us
keep the temperature of the rooms in our homes in a fairly comfortable and steady state.

Likewise, the ANS of our body uses many internal automatic regula-
tors, like thermostats, to maintain a fairly steady state in the inner
world of our body. The ANS controls functions such as:

- Circulation
- Blood pressure and heart rate
- Temperature regulation and perspiration
- Breathing
- Cognition and short-term memory
- Digestion and excretion
- Adapting to an upright physical position (orthostasis)
- Interpretation of external sensory stimuli
- Processing of pain
- Ability to sleep and wake
- Tears and many other "inner world" functions

Autonomic nerves come from the brainstem and spinal cord. Autonomic nerves from the brainstem and sacral spinal cord are parasympathetic nerves. Autonomic nerves from the thoracolumbar spinal cord are sympathetic nerves.

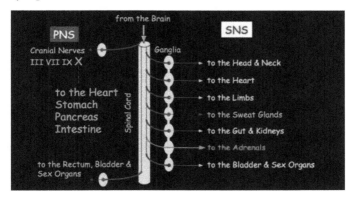

The central nervous system connects to the peripheral nervous system via ganglia that appear like a string of pearls alongside the spinal cord. Preganglionic nerve fibers are myelinated. Postganglionic nerves are non-myelinated. Lesions or damage can occur in

- Preganglionic nerves, as in traumatic brain injury where myelinated nerves are damaged;

- Ganglia, as in autoimmune autonomic ganglionopathy where the immune system attacks the ganglia;

- Postganglionic nerves, as in small fiber neuropathy where small fiber nerves of the peripheral nervous system are damaged or not functioning properly.

Function

The function of the ANS can be divided into three main categories: sympathetic, parasympathetic, and enteric.

The **sympathetic nervous system** is responsible for responding to the stress of daily living and various emergencies. It provides stimulation, when needed, to vital organs and glands by triggering actions, such as increasing heart rate, increasing oxygenation, and producing perspiration.

The ANS can be further divided into the following subsystems:

Subsystems of the Autonomic Nervous System	
Sympathetic	**Like the gas pedal in a car**, adrenaline and other chemical messengers give the body strength to function and fight off danger; blood vessels constrict to push oxygen rich blood to vital organs; airways open, enabling more oxygen rich blood; the heart beats faster and digestion slows when the sympathetic nervous system is engaged or stimulated.
Parasympathetic	**Like the brake pedal in the car**, the body slows down to rest, restore, and digest. Digestive enzymes are released, heart rate slows, blood vessels dilate, airways return to normal, and healing of the body occurs.
Enteric	**The nervous system of the gut** is a mesh-like fabric of neurons (nerve cells) that control the function of the gastrointestinal tract and produce a vast array of chemical messengers essential to the entire nervous system. More norepinephrine, dopamine, and serotonin are produced in the gut than in any other part of the body.

When the ANS is working properly, there is a balance between the gas of the sympathetic nervous system and the brakes of the parasympathetic nervous system. There is also a normal functioning of the gut, which allows proper digestion of food, absorption of nutrients, and release of appropriate chemical messengers of the body. This proper balance between the sympathetic and parasympathetic nervous systems provides a steady inner world or homeostasis.

When this balance is off, the inner world of the body is not in a steady state, and this adversely affects the function of many and/or all organ systems of the body. When the steady state of the inner world is off balance or parts of the ANS are not working, the condition is called dysautonomia.

The **parasympathetic nervous system** is responsible for the restorative needs of the body, including rest, relaxation, and digestion. The ebb and flow of the parasympathetic and sympathetic nervous systems in a normal system acts like waves on the beach and creates a balance between stress and rest in diurnal activities.

The **enteric nervous system** is responsible for the functions of the gastrointestinal system, including motility, absorption of micronutrients, and the release of a wide array of chemical messengers into the body.

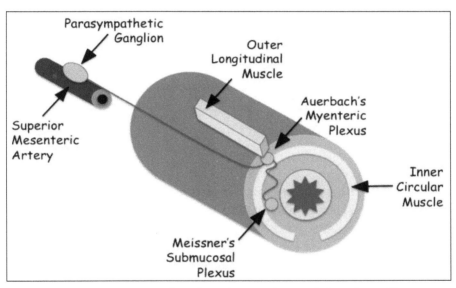

Autonomic neurons are found in plexuses (networks) in the walls. Auerbach's plexus (also called the myenteric plexus) is between the longitudinal and circular layers of smooth muscle; and Meissner's plexus, which is derived from fibers coming from Auerbach's plexus, is in the submucosal layer in the walls of blood vessels. Auerbach's plexus receives parasympathetic and sympathetic innervation. Meissner's plexus receives purely parasympathetic innervation.

7

CHEMICAL MESSENGERS

ADRENALINE—A DOUBLE-EDGED SWORD OF THE INNER WORLD

The energy of the crowd is insane. Twenty thousand people. It's the biggest jolt of adrenaline. It's very hard to explain. You know the old story about the woman lifting the car off her kid? It's in that realm. You can actually hurt yourself and not know it.

Tom Petty, Rock Star
Esquire Magazine Interview
June 29, 2006

One of the most powerful chemical messengers of the autonomic nervous system (ANS) is adrenaline. Also known in scientific communities as epinephrine, when called upon this formidable chemical courses throughout the body via the bloodstream. Adrenaline is derived from noradrenaline, which is also known as norepinephrine.

Adrenaline is secreted in small increments every day, even during the most basic tasks, such as getting out of bed in the morning. During highly stressful moments, adrenaline surges through our bloodstream and enables us to respond to acute stress or danger.

The term "fight or flight response" was first described by Walter B. Cannon in 1915 at Harvard University after observing the natural physical changes that occur, including a surge of adrenaline, in response to life-threatening stress.

The ANS depends on the proper balance of adrenaline in response to both the normal stress of daily living and to the high stress of acute situations. Adrenaline has many physical effects on the body.

7

CHEMICAL MESSENGERS

KEY PLAYERS
OF THE INNER WORLD

A living organism is nothing but a wonderful machine endowed with the most marvelous properties and set going by means of the most complex and delicate mechanism.

Claude Bernard
From *An Introduction to the Study
of Experimental Medicine* (1865),
as translated by Henry Copley Greene (1957)

The chemical mediators of the body are like stars in the sky. They are too numerous to count, and some have yet to be identified. In the study of the autonomic nervous system (ANS) there are specific key players, such as catecholamines, and many auxiliary players, such as histamines, serotonin, prostaglandins, nitric oxide, and endothelins, among others. Here we will focus on the key players, or main chemical messengers of the ANS as they relate to their specific subsystems.

Catecholamines (pronounced cat-a-COLA-mean) are key players in the ANS. Two of the most important catecholamine chemical messengers of the ANS are Norepinephrine (NE) and Epinephrine (EPI). Dopamine is another catecholamine that has an effect on the ANS. Dopamine, norepinephrine, and epinephrine are like the grandmother, mother, and daughter in a small chemical family. Epinephrine (adrenaline) is derived from norepinephrine, and norepinephrine is derived from dopamine (Learn more about catecholamines in "The Principles of Autonomic Medicine" by David S. Goldstein, at *www.TheDysautonomiaProject/Resources/2*).

It can:

- Increase blood pressure
- Increase heart rate
- Increase blood flow to the muscles of the body
- Expand airways in the lungs
- Enlarge pupils of the eyes for better sight
- Decrease blood flow to the gut
- Cause a metabolic change to maximize blood glucose/energy levels throughout the body

Mom Lifts Car to Save Son

Mrs. Maxwell Rogers, a resident of Tampa, Florida, earned a Guinness World record by lifting one end of a station wagon after the car fell off a bumper jack and onto her teenage son on April 24, 1960. During the amazing car lift, fueled by an unusual burst of adrenaline, Mrs. Rogers, who weighed 123 lbs., lifted an estimated 1000 lbs. and sustained fractures of several vertebrae.[1]

This is one of many reports of people using supernatural strength in life-threatening situations. Although Mrs. Rogers was severely injured, it is likely she did not sense pain at the time because the adrenaline that flooded her body has the ability to block pain receptors that normally protect us from injury.

Addicted to Adrenaline?

Although adrenaline is a natural chemical that is essential for functioning, many people are drawn to activities that give them an extra boost of this neurotransmitter. Exercise is great activity that boosts a healthy increase of both adrenaline and norepinephrine in the bloodstream. But, what happens when we have repeated surges in adrenaline when there is no real danger or stress? And why is it that many people today who live high stress lives also choose recreational activities that cause additional adrenaline surges?

Movie producers seem to know this addiction well, as a vast majority of films are action-packed thrillers that are expected to give us an

---

[1] Smith, Jack. "Guinness Gives Records." Tuscaloosa News, April 3, 1968.

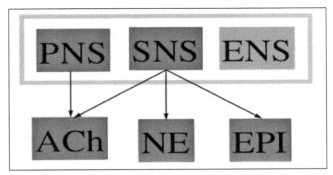

The parasympathetic and sympathetic nervous systems and their specific chemical messengers. The enteric nervous system has many chemical messengers.

The sympathetic nervous system has three components or subsystems, and each can be recognized by its main chemical messenger.

The sympathetic noradrenergic nervous system consists mainly of thin, slow-conducting, non-myelinated, post-ganglionic nerves. Although the neurotransmitter mediating the ganglionic transmission is acetylcholine, acting at nicotinic receptors, the main chemical messenger of the sympathetic noradrenergic nervous system is norepinephrine (NE). This neurotransmitter is released from the post-ganglionic nerve terminals.

Perhaps the most prominent effect of this part of the sympathetic nervous system is constriction of blood vessels—especially of arterioles, thus reducing total peripheral resistance to blood flow in the body. Blood flow is also decreased to the gut, skeletal muscles, and kidneys. Blood flow to vital organs is generally preserved. Stimulation also causes the pupils to dilate, skin pallor, and the salivary glands to secrete thick saliva. The force and rate of the heartbeat increase. Smooth muscle cells in the 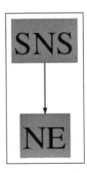 airways relax. The hair stands up because of stimulation of arrector pili muscles in the skin. In the kidneys, norepinephrine promotes tubular reabsorption of sodium.

Norepinephrine exerts these effects mainly by stimulating alpha-adrenoceptors. It also is an agonist at beta-1 adrenoceptors, but unlike adrenaline, norepinephrine is a relatively poor agonist at beta-2 adrenoceptors. Norepinephrine is a neurotransmitter, not a hormone. Its

adrenaline rush even though we're just sitting and watching. On *You-Tube* you can watch a back-to-back showing of trailers from the top 20 movies that fuel our adrenaline, from *The Dark Knight* to *The Fast and the Furious*.

When our Lives are Filled with Chronic Stress

According to the Mayo Clinic, long-term chronic stress may put your health at risk. "The body's stress-response system is usually self-limiting. Once a perceived threat has passed, hormone levels return to normal. As adrenaline and cortisol levels drop, your heart rate and blood pressure return to baseline levels, and other systems resume their regular activities. But when stressors are always present and you constantly feel under attack, that fight-or-flight reaction stays turned on.

The long-term activation of the stress-response system—and the subsequent overexposure to cortisol and other stress hormones—can disrupt almost all your body's processes. This puts you at increased risk of numerous health problems."[2]

Since adrenaline is the most powerful chemical messenger of the ANS, it may be helpful to think of it as a double-edged sword:

- Essential for healthy living; but,
- Capable of causing harm when overused.

In dysautonomias, acute or chronic stress is a common trigger for onset or relapse of symptoms. This will be discussed further in Chapter 26, "Top Enemies of Dysautonomia."

---

[2] Mayo Clinic Staff. Patient Care & Health Information; Healthy Lifestyle Stress Management. *www.mayoclinic.org*, July, 2015.

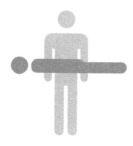

effects in the body are determined mainly by it reaching adrenoceptors before it reaches the bloodstream.

The **sympathetic adrenergic nervous system**, or adrenomedullary hormonal system, regulates "emergency" processes, such as perceived or anticipated threats to overall homeostasis, lack of essential fuels (glucose and oxygen), inadequate blood flow to vital organs, and hostile encounters. In such emergencies, adrenaline (synonymous with epinephrine, EPI) is released from the adrenal glands. Adrenaline is the main chemical messenger of the sympathetic adrenergic nervous system.

The connection from the spinal cord to the adrenal medullary cells is direct, via myelinated fibers, so the adrenal medulla can release adrenaline into the bloodstream rapidly, as needed in sudden emergencies. Cortisol, the main steroid of the adrenal cortex, is a trophic factor for PNMT, the enzyme that converts norepinephrine to adrenaline. While norepinephrine is a neurotransmitter that is released in the nerve terminals and acts locally, adrenaline is a hormone that is released into the bloodstream and then distributed widely throughout the body.

Adrenaline stimulates all types of adrenoceptors. Because of stimulation of beta-2 adrenoceptors on vascular smooth muscle cells, adrenaline increases blood flow to skeletal muscle. At higher concentrations, adrenaline produces stimulation of the heart by increasing both the rate and force of contraction, 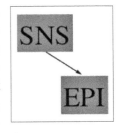 and it constricts blood vessels by stimulating alpha-adrenoceptors. Adrenaline also causes pallor, relaxes the gut, increases sweating, increases core temperature, and increases glucose levels. Failure of the sympathetic adrenergic system can cause a tendency to low glucose levels (hypoglycemia).

The **sympathetic cholinergic nervous system** consists mainly of thin, slow-conducting, non-myelinated post-ganglionic nerves. The neurotransmitter mediating the ganglionic transmission is acetylcholine, acting at nicotinic receptors. The neurotransmitter released 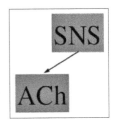 from the post-ganglionic nerve terminals, as the main

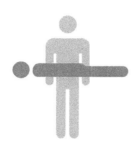

chemical messenger of this part of the sympathetic nervous system, is the neurotransmitter acetylcholine (ACh).

The sympathetic cholinergic nervous system acts on sweat glands that mediate thermoregulatory, gustatory, and emotional responses in the body. It is the component of the sympathetic nervous system that plays a major role in sweating, such as when you perspire upon exposure to high temperatures, or when your forehead breaks out in sweat after eating spicy foods, or when your palms or armpits get wet during an emotionally upsetting event.

The **Parasympathetic nervous system (PNS)** in many ways acts like the opposite of an emergency system. "Vegetative" behaviors, and activities that increase instead of use up energy are associated with increased activity of this system. Examples are sleeping, eating, salivating, digesting, and excreting waste.

Most parasympathetic nerves are cranial nerves in the brainstem. These nerves travel to many parts of the body, including the eyes, face, tongue, heart, and most of the gastrointestinal system. The vagus nerve, or tenth cranial nerve, is the most widely used nerve of the PNS. Connected to several places inside the chest, abdomen, and pelvis, stimulation of the vagus nerve decreases hart rate and increases smooth muscle tone, mucus secretion in 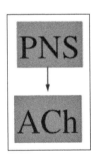 in the airways, and secretion of stomach acid and digestive hormones. Additional parasympathetic nerves are found in the sacral region of the spinal cord, which travel to the genital organs, urinary bladder, and lower gastrointestinal tract. In parasympathetic nerves, the ganglia are located close to or even inside the target organs, and so the post-ganglionic, non-myelinated neurons are short.

The neurotransmitter at all the autonomic ganglia is acetylcholine. Acetylcholine binds to nicotinic receptors on the cell bodies of the post-ganglionic nerves, and is released from the post-ganglionic nerve terminals in the target organs where the receptors in the target organs are muscarinic. Acetylcholine is the main chemical messenger of the PNS.

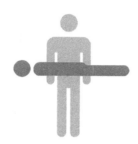

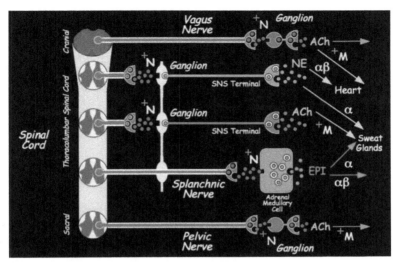

An overview of the distribution of sympathetic and parasympathetic nerves.

The **Enteric nervous system (ENS)** produces numerous chemical messengers that affect the autonomic nervous system. Autonomic neurons are found in plexuses (networks) in the walls of the gastrointestinal tract, as shown in the diagram at the end of the previous chapter.

The ENS includes not only autonomic fibers but also intrinsic neuronal cells called ganglion cells. The ganglion cells migrate from the neural crest during fetal development and are required for movement of intestinal contents. The ENS contains many neurotransmitters. It is a surprising fact that most of the norepinephrine, dopamine, and serotonin made in the body is synthesized in the gut.

Measuring Chemical Messengers

Measuring levels of catecholamines and related chemicals is a key part of the workup of many patients with dysautonomias, as these are the only main chemical messengers of the autonomic nervous system that can be measured in body fluids such as plasma, urine, or spinal fluid.

Drugs that affect the production, release, or inactivation of catecholamines, or that work by stimulating or blocking receptors for catecholamines, are mainstays in the treatment of various forms of dysautonomia. Directly or indirectly, virtually every dysautonomia and every treatment for dysautonomias involves catecholamines.

8

THE DYSAUTONOMIA UNIVERSE

HOW ARE DYSAUTONOMIAS CLASSIFIED?

Dysautonomia is a general term that describes any disorder of the autonomic (automatic) nervous system (ANS). These disorders usually involve abnormal symptoms in many organ systems, including cardiac, gastrointestinal, neurological, and pulmonary, as well as others. Dysautonomias can range from mild to disabling, and some are life threatening.

Since there are many forms of dysautonomia, we use the singular term "dysautonomia" to reference dysautonomia in general or when referring to one specific condition, such as orthostatic hypotension. We use "dysautonomias," plural, when referring to many disorders of the ANS.

> *A person with dysautonomia often does not look sick on the outside, but can be very unwell on the inside.*

When in Life do Dysautonomias Occur?

Dysautonomias can appear at any age in the life cycle and can be categorized by when in life they appear.

1. **Early pediatric:** highly genetic / occurs during development, as in familial dysautonomia;

2. **Late pediatric-adult:** functional deficits / usually dysfunction of the ANS, as in postural orthostatic tachycardia syndrome (POTS);

3. **Geriatric:** often neurodegenerative / usually failure of the ANS, as in multiple system atrophy (MSA) or pure autonomic failure (PAF).

8

THE DYSAUTONOMIA UNIVERSE

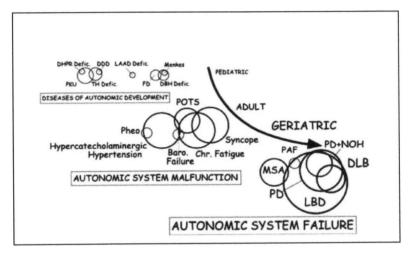

Illustrated by David S. Goldstein, MD, PhD

There are many forms of dysautonomia, which can occur at any age--pediatric, adult, and/or geriatric.

Pediatric

In infants and children, dysautonomias often reflect problems in the development of the autonomic nervous system. Frequently the cause is a genetic change, mutation. One type of mutation, found in people of Ashkenazi extraction, causes familial dysautonomia. Another mutation produces dysautonomias in children because of a type of phenylketonuria (PKU). Other causes include "kinky hair disease" (Menkes disease), and in Hirschsprung's disease there is a lack of development of nerve cells of the enteric nervous system in the colon. There are also genetic diseases of proteins required for synthesizing or storing catecholamines. In general, dysautonomias in early childhood are rare.

What Does Dysautonomia Look Like?

Dysautonomias involve disorders of the "inner world" or automatic functions of the body. As a result, a person with dysautonomia often does not look sick on the outside; but they can be very unwell on the inside. The exception to this would be if the dysautonomia is secondary to another condition (such as Parkinson's disease) involving loss of somatic (voluntary) muscle tone, or another illness with "outer world" symptoms. This is why dysautonomia is easily misdiagnosed and sometimes referred to as an invisible illness.

Autonomic Dysfunction vs. Autonomic Failure

Dysautonomias can also be categorized by the way the ANS is currently working. When the autonomic nerves and normal reflexes of those nerves are active, but not working correctly, this is considered a "dysfunction" of the ANS. When the nerves are damaged, or not working at all, this is considered "failure." Testing of the autonomic reflexes may be helpful in distinguishing between autonomic dysfunction vs. failure. In some cases, especially those involving younger patients, nerves can be restored and healed. In most cases, conditions involving autonomic failure are neurodegenerative, meaning the nerves are gradually losing their ability to work.

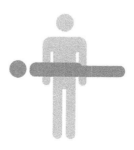

Adult

In teens and adults, dysautonomias usually reflect functional changes in a generally intact autonomic nervous system. Examples are autonomic syncope (also called neurally mediated syncope, vasovagal syncope, or neurocardiogenic syncope), in which the person suffers from frequent episodes of fainting, or near fainting; postural tachycardia syndrome, in which the person cannot tolerate standing up for long periods and has a rapid pulse rate during standing; and hypernoradrenergic hypertension, in which overactivity of the sympathetic noradrenergic system causes a form of high blood pressure.

Dysautonomias in adults often are associated with—and may be secondary to—another disease process or a drug. Common secondary causes include medications, diabetes (diabetic autonomic neuropathy, or DAN), chemotherapy for cancer, irradiation of the neck, and alcoholism. Less commonly, activities of components of the autonomic nervous system change in an attempt to compensate for dehydration or low blood volume, or when a viral infection impacts the autonomic nervous system, or when the body attacks itself (as in autoimmune autonomic ganglionopathy, or AAG).

Geriatric

In the elderly, dysautonomia typically reflects a neurodegenerative disease. The degeneration may be in the form of lesions in the central nervous system, as in multiple system atrophy, or in loss of autonomic nerves, as in Parkinson disease. Most geriatric cases involve damage to the nerves that results in loss of autonomic reflexes, also known as autonomic failure.

See page 103 for a list of abnormal responses in blood pressure and heart rate upon standing.

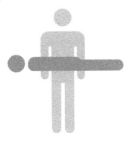

9

ORTHOSTATIC INTOLERANCE SPECTRUM

LIVING WITH ORTHOSTATIC INTOLERANCE

You'll be doing everything right, and then all of the sudden you start to feel really bad. Give in to it. Lie down. Don't try to push through it. If you do, you'll make your symptoms worse.

Randy Thompson, MD

Only about 40% of people with dysautonomia actually pass out, but 99% have overwhelming fatigue. Most patients have daily symptoms that they learn to live with and episodes where the symptoms become overwhelming and they need to lie down. Lying down relieves orthostatic stress and improves symptoms in orthostatic intolerance. Most patients have many symptoms beyond lightheadedness. Take a look and see if any of these other symptoms are familiar to you.

Common Symptoms Reported by Patients with Orthostatic Intolerance

Lightheadedness	Fainting	Fatigue
Brain Fog / Mental Clouding	Difficulty finding words	Short-term Memory Loss
Sensory Hypersensitivities (e.g. light, sound, motion, touch)	Paresthesias (pins and needles feeling)	Numbness of hands and feet
Coat Hanger Pain in neck and shoulders	Migraine Headaches	Other Headaches

9

ORTHOSTATIC INTOLERANCE SPECTRUM

MANAGING ORTHOSTATIC INTOLERANCE

A major way dysautonomias cause problems is by producing orthostatic intolerance (OI). Patients with OI cannot tolerate prolonged standing.

Orthostatic intolerance is not a diagnosis. It is a state of being that involves many symptoms, including dizziness or lightheadedness while standing. Understanding a few basics about OI may help in treating the patient and making decisions about the cause of a specific case or disease.

OI is seen in many different conditions, including dysautonomias. About 60% of patients with chronic fatigue syndrome have chronic orthostatic intolerance, along with postural tachycardia syndrome (POTS) or autonomically mediated syncope* (fainting), or both.

The fact that there are many possible causes of orthostatic intolerance poses a challenge to any doctor trying to come up with a diagnosis to explain orthostatic intolerance in a particular patient. The Orthostatic Intolerance Spectrum may help the new practitioner in managing orthostatic intolerance. It is divided into three sectors: episodic OI, chronic OI, and neurocirculatory failure. A starting point in identifying a cause of orthostatic intolerance is to answer this question: In which tri-sector of the Orthostatic Intolerance Spectrum does the patient fall? (See diagram next page.)

Episodic OI

Episodic OI means the difficulty in standing does not occur consistently enough to warrant ongoing clinical management. Dehydration, stress

---

* "Autonomically mediated syncope" is used throughout this book to describe syncope that involves dysfunction of the autonomic nervous system. This condition is also known as neurocardiogenic syncope, vasovagal syncope, and neurally mediated syncope.

Exercise Intolerance	Heat Intolerance	Abnormal Sweating
Temperature Dysregulation	Abdominal Pain	Nausea
Vomiting	Constipation	Diarrhea
Gastroparesis (Gastrointestinal tract stops moving)	Palpitations	Chest Pain
Difficulty Breathing	Anxiety or Depression	Difficulty with depth perception
Tinnitus (Ear ringing)	Flushing (dry, red, hot face or upper body)	Cyanosis in feet (bluish/purple color change)

Plans Will Change

You'll make plans to go out with friends and, just before it's time to go, you start to feel bad. Since your episodes will start with symptoms of feeling bad, it's important for you to pay attention to your body. What kind of "bad feeling" or first symptoms do you experience? It's important to note differences like those between being tired and being fatigued. (See Chapter 10 for more about the difference.) Your symptoms may vary, but after time you may begin to recognize a helpful pattern. Once you realize that you are starting to become symptomatic, give in to it. Lie down and rest. The relief of orthostatic (upright) stress will improve your symptoms.

Once you get into an episode, it may be helpful to load up on fluids and salt. Drinking 32 oz. of cool liquids quickly, along with eating a salty snack, may help speed your recovery. Most important is to pay attention to your body and, when you start to feel bad, change your plans and recover before your symptoms worsen.

Brain Fog—A Difficult Symptom for Most People to Understand

Brain fog, or mental clouding, occurs when there is not an ideal amount of blood flow to the cerebral cortex (not a dangerously low level but a smaller than normal amount). This lower blood flow causes difficulties with concentrating, finding words, laying down short-term memory

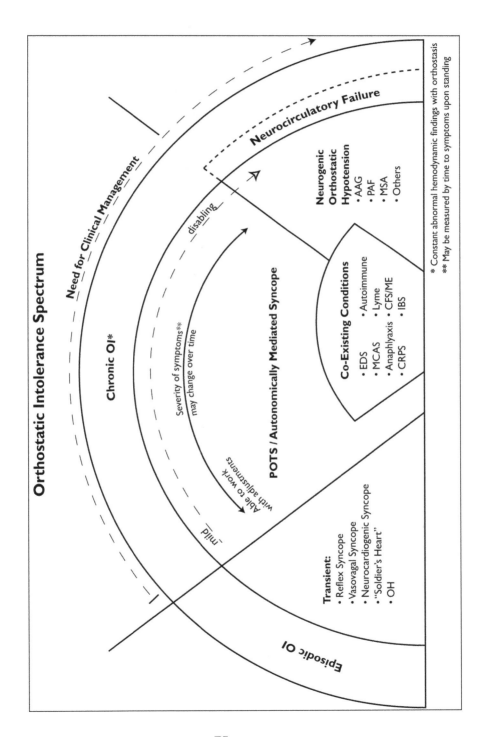

Orthostatic Intolerance Spectrum

Need for Clinical Management

Neurocirculatory Failure

Chronic OI*

disabling

Severity of symptoms**
may change over time

POTS / Autonomically Mediated Syncope

Able to work
with adjustments

mild

Neurogenic Orthostatic Hypotension
- AAG
- PAF
- MSA
- Others

Co-Existing Conditions
- EDS
- MCAS
- Anaphlyaxis
- CRPS
- Autoimmune
- Lyme
- CFS/ME
- IBS

Transient:
- Reflex Syncope
- Vasovagal Syncope
- Neurocardiogenic Syncope
- "Soldier's Heart"
- OH

Episodic OI

* Constant abnormal hemodynamic findings with orthostasis
** May be measured by time to symptoms upon standing

tracks, and other symptoms. Don't worry, you are not losing IQ points. It is a temporary symptom that can improve when you reduce stress and get good rest.

Learn more about Brain Fog in Chapter 13 by Dr. Julian Stewart.

It is important to note that sitting upright is an orthostatic position which may cause you to experience symptoms. It is helpful to determine how long you can stand and/or sit upright before experiencing symptoms, so that you can be prepared and plan activities appropriately.

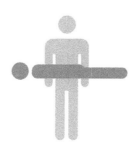

prolonged bed rest, or illness may cause this occasional faint, or drop in blood pressure. This occasional problem is a normal reaction to an abnormal flow of blood in a person with a healthy autonomic nervous system and must be differentiated from more serious conditions. This is an important sector for the physician to understand because it is easy to make the mistake of diagnosing a patient with a relatively benign case of episodic OI and miss the warning signs of a more serious condition requiring ongoing clinical management. Therefore, the consistency in abnormal blood pressure and heart rate must be determined prior to diagnosis.

Chronic OI

Most dysautonomia patients fall into this category, which explains why this trisection is proportionally larger. In chronic OI the severity of symptoms may fluctuate over time, but the patient consistently experiences symptoms and demonstrates abnormal drops in blood pressure or abnormal increases in heart rate, or both, upon standing. The severity of symptoms can range from mild to disabling, and can often be correlated with the amount of time that passes before the patient becomes symptomatic. In mild cases, the patient may be able to stand for many minutes using counter maneuvers; in more severe cases, the patient may be able to stand for less than a minute before experiencing symptoms. In chronic OI, the person does not have sympathetic neurocirculatory failure, as the blood pressure does not fall consistently when the person stands up (although the person can have delayed orthostatic hypotension after many minutes of standing). Instead, even though the person's blood pressure is maintained for a period of time during standing, the person still feels dizzy or lightheaded, and often experiences additional symptoms.

The assortment of symptoms beyond lightheadedness that patients often experience may involve many or all organ systems. These symptoms include nausea, visual disturbances, headache, leg pain, brain fog, and more. The severity of symptoms may change over time and worsen with external stress, including emotional stress, physical stress, or pain.

Common dysautonomias involving chronic OI are postural orthostatic tachycardia syndrome (POTS) and autonomically mediated syncope.

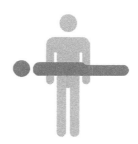

In this patient population, identifying the exact condition is not as important as working with patients to help them understand and manage their condition with the aim of improving function. Treatment options are similar for this cohort of patients. As a clinician, it is important to:

- Note the need for clinical management generally increases with symptom severity;

- Determine if chronic OI is part of a primary problem or if it is part of a compensatory reaction to something else;

- Consider possible coexisting conditions;

- Realize that patients who initially have mild symptoms can quickly become disabled by a lack of proper management and the presence of pain and/or stress. (Thus patients with mild cases need to be cautioned to watch for warning signs and be educated about what to do if their symptoms worsen.) With good management, usually with trial and error of various treatments over time, symptoms can improve.

- The aim of treatment in patients with chronic OI is to improve function.

Neurocirculatory Failure

In this form of orthostatic intolerance there is failure of the sympathetic nervous system to correctly regulate the heart and blood vessels. We call this sympathetic neurocirculatory failure. In dysautonomias that produce sympathetic neurocirculatory failure, the patient consistently has a fall in blood pressure during standing. Some conditions involving neurocirculatory failure are Parkinson's disease with neurogenic orthostatic hypotension (PD-OH), pure autonomic failure (PAF), and autoimmune autonomic ganglionopathy (AAG).

Most cases of neurocirculatory failure are neurodegenerative in nature, and for these, the aim of treatment is to slow the neurodegenerative process and treat symptoms. In some cases, especially if the patient is young, healing of the damaged nerves can occur over time. In these cases, unlike in cases involving chronic OI, it is very helpful to understand the specific condition and mechanisms involved in the dysautonomia in order to provide proper treatment, because sometimes an exact diagnosis can lead to a very specific and effective treatment.

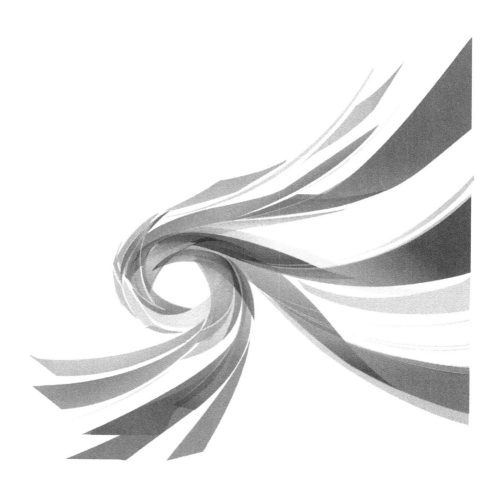

SECTION 3

Assessment & Diagnosis

Today, the Average Patient Waits Approximately Six Years to be Diagnosed

My daughter has been chronically ill for years. I can't count the number of doctors we've had consult on her case. As I listened to the presentation tonight I was blown away. I realized she has dysautonomia.

Tony Degina
CEO, HCA Largo Medical Center
After attending The Dysautonomia Project's
VIP Kick Off Dinner Party, October 9, 2014

10

CLUES IT MIGHT BE DYAUTONOMIA

DO YOU HAVE THESE TWO SYMPTOMS?

Many dysautonomia patients have these two symptoms in common:

1. Difficulty standing still for long periods of time.

Most people don't pay close attention to this important clue that may be a sign of orthostatic intolerance. Some patients with dysautonomia are unaware they have a difficulty standing still because they have unconsciously developed habits or counter maneuvers (see more about counter maneuvers in Chapter 30).

Here are a few questions to ask yourself about your comfort with standing still:

- Are you able to stand still (without moving) for thirty minutes at a time without difficulty?
- When standing, whether talking with people or standing in long lines, do you find yourself fidgeting and/or constantly moving your body around (e.g. moving or tapping feet, swaying) more than most people?
- Do you get lightheaded after standing up quickly?

One doctor on The Dysautonomia Project's International Medical Advisory Board says he can go to the Walmart store near his office, watch the people standing in line, and make a pretty accurate prediction about who his next patients will be.

10

CLUES IT MIGHT BE DYAUTONOMIA

THE TOP SEVEN SIGNS AND SYMPTOMS

There is a strong chance you have already seen many patients with dysautonomia. But, because it is not well taught in medical education today, and because its presentation is widely heterogeneous, most patients with dysautonomia remain undiagnosed.

While this list may be helpful for initially recognizing dysautonomias, it merely scratches the surface of the wide array of common patient complaints. It is important to note that in up to 25% of the cases, the patient's chief complaint is not included in this list.

7 Signs and Symptoms:

1. Difficulty Standing Still
2. Fatigue
3. Lightheadedness
4. Nausea and Other GI Symptoms
5. Brain Fog or Mental Clouding
6. Palpitations, Chest Discomfort
7. Shortness of Breath or Difficulty Breathing

If your patient has chronic health problems, it may be worthwhile to ask if they have experienced any of the symptoms on this list. If so, a comprehensive clinical assessment that focuses on the autonomic nervous

2. Fatigue

Everyone gets tired. Not everyone experiences fatigue. For most fatigue sufferers the symptom waxes and wanes. For a few, it is a constant companion. Unfortunately, most people don't know there is a difference between being tired and being fatigued. From a medical standpoint, this is the difference between a diagnosis of "normal" and "abnormal."

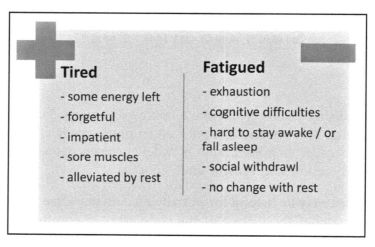

Tired

- some energy left
- forgetful
- impatient
- sore muscles
- alleviated by rest

Fatigued

- exhaustion
- cognitive difficulties
- hard to stay awake / or fall asleep
- social withdrawl
- no change with rest

When you are tired you may be forgetful, impatient, and have muscle soreness; but, you still have some energy left, and rest alleviates the symptoms. When your body is fatigued, there is no energy beyond what your body uses for survival. Common symptoms include cognitive difficulties, anxiety, difficulty staying awake, difficulty falling asleep, and you avoid social activities that used to create enjoyment.

It is important to keep in mind that the absence of both of these symptoms does not mean that you do not have a disorder of the autonomic nervous system. Ruling out ANS disorders needs to be done by an educated physician. However, if you have both of these symptoms, ask your doctor about dysautonomia.

system may be worthwhile (see "The Principles of Autonomic Medicine" for a list of top signs and symptoms based on the various components of the autonomic nervous system. *www.TheDysautonomiaProject. org/Resources/2*).

Symptoms and signs of dysautonomias result from alterations in activities of one or more components of the autonomic nervous system. Activation or inhibition of the different components of the autonomic nervous system produces different effects on the body.

The Mayo Clinic Autonomic Laboratory assesses autonomic severity based on the results of their assessment in six categories.

Six Domains of Compass 31*: An Assessment Tool for Identifying Symptom Severity in Autonomic Nervous System Dysfunction

1. Orthostatic Intolerance (difficulty sitting or standing upright)

2. Gastrointestinal (difficulty related to digestion)

3. Vasomotor (abnormal blood vessel functioning)

4. Secretomotor (difficulty with sweating, tearing, and other fluid production)

5. Bladder (difficulty with urine excretion)

6. Pupilomotor (difficulty with eyes and/or vision)

* Sletten, et al., Mayo Clinic Proceedings; Volume 87, Issue 12, Pages 1196-1201, December 2012

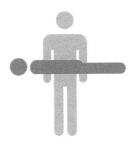

11

ASSESSMENT IN THE CLINIC

COME PREPARED

The patient is the best expert when it comes to helping me diagnose the condition.

Jan K. Cornelius, DDS

If you are reading this book, it is likely you already know that when it comes to treating patients with dysautonomia there are two types of doctors:

1. Doctors who are educated about dysautonomia;
2. Doctors who are not.

If your doctor knows something about dysautonomia, he or she will likely use some variation of the assessment process that follows.

If the doctor is not educated about dysautonomia, it is up to you to determine: Is this doctor willing to learn about dysautonomia and work with me to improve my health? If the answer is yes, then bring your physician information about dysautonomia and any information you have about your specific case that might help in determining a correct diagnosis. It may also be helpful to bring a copy of this book to share with your physician to facilitate a more meaningful discussion.

> *If the doctor is not educated about dysautonomia, it is up to you to determine: Is this doctor willing to learn about dysautonomia and work with me to improve my health?*

If the answer is no, don't be discouraged. Since this condition is not well taught in medical education, it is common to meet doctors who are not familiar with dysautonomias and don't have time right now to learn about them. If you find yourself in this situation, change doctors.

11

ASSESSMENT IN THE CLINIC

THE MOST IMPORTANT MEASURE OF ALL

Initial Diagnostic Criteria

There are two diagnostic criteria for dysautonomia:

1. Clinical assessment, including a comprehensive medical history and physical exam;

2. An Orthostatic Vitals Test and/or other autonomic function test, providing clinical evidence supporting a diagnosis of dysautonomia.

Most important in the evaluation of dysautonomia is the medical history, which consists of several parts. These include the Chief Complaint, the History of the Present Illness (HPI), the Past History, the Family History, the Personal and Social History, and the Review of Systems (ROS). Additional parts of the clinical assessment include a physical exam and, if dysautonomia is suspected, an orthostatic vitals test. Each of these parts is important for diagnosing and managing dysautonomias, but the key component is the HPI. Taking the medical history, especially the HPI, is a skill that must be developed. (See Chapter 12 for more about developing this skill.) A complete listing of all prescribed medications, over-the-counter medications, herbal remedies, and dietary supplements is a key part of the medical history, not only because these can affect autonomic function but also because they can interact to produce unexpected, serious, adverse events.

Determine Sequence of Events

In obtaining the history of the present illness (HPI), one of the most important skills a clinician can acquire is the ability to get the sequence right. A good question to start with is "When was the last time

(For more information, see the upcoming chapter about finding a good primary care doctor.)

When you meet with your doctor you can expect them to spend time asking you questions about your health history, including symptoms and signs of your current health condition. Symptoms are feelings or experiences that you report to the doctor as part of the medical history. Signs are medical findings that a doctor detects during a physical examination or other test.

It is helpful to come prepared with:

- A complete list of symptoms
- Questions you have
- Loose-fitting, comfortable clothing
- Copies of previous medical records (if available)

The physician will ask questions about your health history and current symptoms, will conduct a physical exam, and may conduct an orthostatic vitals test as a part of the initial assessment process.

It is important to note that many physicians have limited time planned for each appointment. Since diagnosing dysautonomia is much more complex than diagnosing localized or acute conditions, such as a kidney stone, a urinary tract infection, or the flu, gathering all the information a physician needs to make a proper assessment may take more time than is allotted in their schedule. You may be asked to come back for a follow-up appointment or individualized testing to complete the initial assessment process.

After the initial assessment, your physician will help determine if further testing is needed.

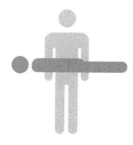

you felt perfectly healthy?" Some dysautonomias develop in a rather stereotypical sequence. An example is a type of autonomic failure known as the cerebellar form of multiple system atrophy (MSA-C) in a man. Men with MSA-C typically relate that the first thing to go wrong, in retrospect, was erectile failure. However, in most males with central neurodegeneration and orthostatic hypotension, the absence of erectile failure as an early finding usually rules out MSA-C. The erectile failure is typically followed by urinary problems—especially urinary retention, eventually to the point of requiring self-catheterization. Then comes slurred speech, a wide-based unsteady gait, and lightheadedness when standing.

What Provokes or Improves Symptoms?

In obtaining the details about symptoms of dysautonomias, it is also important to determine which situations make things worse and which make things better. For instance, patients with neurogenic orthostatic hypotension often relate that their symptoms are worse in the morning, upon heat exposure, after eating a large meal, or after exercise.

Explore Related Symptoms

Because of associations of autonomic failure with non-motor aspects of Lewy body diseases such as Parkinson disease and pure autonomic failure, it is important to ask about whether the patient smells things like other people, sees things like other people, and has any problems with sleep. The clinician is looking for evidence of olfactory dysfunction, visual hallucinations, and dream enactment behavior.

In patients with possible postural tachycardia syndrome (POTS), it is valuable to ask about whether the patient has "double-jointedness" or flushing, since these can be clues to the existence of a coexisting conditions, such as Ehlers-Danlos syndrome and/or mast cell activation disorders.

Subacute development of orthostatic intolerance after a viral illness suggests an autoimmune component of the pathophysiology, whereas a history of frequent fainting or "seizures" since childhood points more to a congenital, genetic component. In a patient with labile blood pressure and orthostatic intolerance, a remote history of irradiation of the neck may suggest the possibility of arterial baroreflex failure due to accelerated arteriosclerosis of the carotid sinus area.

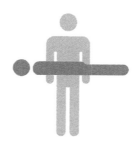

Query Components of the ANS

In patients with orthostatic intolerance or orthostatic hypotension, standing upright can result in an annoying pain in the back of the neck and along the shoulders. Because of the distribution of the discomfort, this is sometimes referred to as the coat hanger sign or coat hanger phenomenon. The "coat hanger phenomenon" refers to pain in the back of the neck during standing. The exact mechanism of the coat hanger phenomenon is unknown, but one theory suggests it is a kind of cramp caused when the anti-gravity muscles holding up the head receive too little blood flow.

> *The "coat hanger phenomenon" refers to pain in the back of the neck during standing.*

It is common for a patient with orthostatic intolerance to bring a bottle of water to the clinical encounter and sip from it periodically as the history is taken. The patients often report that although drinking water continuously doesn't eliminate the symptoms, not drinking water rapidly makes them worse. This may be a clue as to the pathophysiology of chronic orthostatic intolerance. Perhaps the kidneys are less efficient in reabsorbing filtered water, and the water bottle sign is part of a behavioral compensation. It might be worth looking into whether there is a problem with aquaporins or with vasopressin, the anti-diuretic hormone that is the main water retention hormone of the body, in patients with chronic orthostatic intolerance and the water bottle sign.

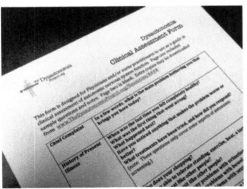

The Clinical Assessment Form is a tool that can be used by physicians and nurse practitioners to guide the assessment process in the clinic. If dysautonomia is suspected, an orthostatic vitals test may be performed by a member of the nursing staff or other health professional in the clinic to give the practitioner hemodynamic data that occurs upon orthostatic stress. (See Chapter 14 for more on the usefulness of orthostatic vitals in clinical assessment.)

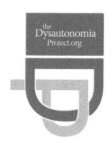

12

OBTAINING THE HISTORY OF THE PRESENT ILLNESS

AN IMPORTANT SKILL

by David S. Goldstein, MD, PhD, and Co-Author

I take what the patient says as gospel. The patient knows best how he or she feels, and in my experience patients always tell the truth.

Taking the medical history, obtaining the history of the present illness (HPI), is a skill that must be honed by learning and experience, ideally under the direct supervision of a mentor.

I usually start by asking the patient, "When was the last time you felt perfectly healthy?" It's amazing learning the answers, which can range from "I've never been healthy." to "I was fine until..." to "It was such a gradual thing, I don't know."

My screening questions generally query each of the components of the autonomic nervous system. The questions are designed not to be leading. For instance, about sympathetic cholinergic function, I ask, "Do you sweat like other people?" About sympathetic noradrenergic function, I ask, "Are you able to tolerate standing still?" About parasympathetic cholinergic function, I ask, "Are you able to make spit and tears like other people? Have you noticed anything different about how your GI system is working? Have you noticed anything different about your urination?" In a man I also ask, "Are you able to have an erection and ejaculate?" Depending on the specific conditions I have in mind, I also ask questions related to dysautonomia syndromes.

Most patients with orthostatic intolerance are women. At the risk of seeming chauvinistic, my main screening question for a woman referred for orthostatic intolerance is, "Who does your shopping?"

If the answer is, "I do. I love to shop." then that is the end of my line of questioning. A positive answer is something like, "Well, not me." When I ask, "Why not?" the answer I'm looking for is, "Because I can't tolerate standing still in line. I start to feel faint or lightheaded or weak, or I have to twist my legs like a pretzel, or I have to sit down."

Each of the parts of the medical history is important for diagnosing and managing dysautonomias, but the key component is the (HPI).

The HPI is basically a narrative of the condition. It is best to obtain the HPI from the patient directly. There are records to review of hospitalizations, test results, and previous accounts of the medical history and physical examination (HPE). These are all subject to mistakes and often are uninformative. The patient's story of his or her symptoms, especially with the help of family or significant others, is at least as likely to be correct and informative.

Unfortunately, this key aspect of the medical encounter is not reimbursed adequately considering its importance and the time and effort involved.

Some aspects of the screening autonomic history

Chief Complaint: In a few words, what's the main problem bothering you that brings you here today?
HPI: When was the last time you felt completely healthy? What was the first thing that went wrong? What happened next? Have you noticed anything that makes the problem worse or better? What treatments have been tried, and how did you respond?
Autonomic Review of Systems: Who does your shopping? Are you able to tolerate standing, exercise, heat, a large meal? Do you sweat like other people? Do you make spit like other people? Have you noticed any problems with urination? Have you noticed any problems with bowel movements? Have you noticed any problems with sexual function?

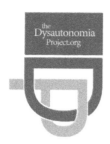

13

WHAT IS BRAIN FOG?

by Julian Stewart, MD, PhD

"Brain Fog" is a common complaint in patients with POTS. Patients often use the term to describe symptoms of lightheadedness, impaired awareness, mental fatigue, and cognitive deficits.[1] Although the constellation of symptoms is imprecise, and has until recently lacked clear physiological correlates, there is evidence that brain fog is closely associated with upright posture in POTS and is related to specific abnormalities found in cerebral blood flow (CBF).

At first it was hypothesized that orthostatic reduction in mean CBF was the culprit. While on average CBF does decrease excessively in POTS,[2] later scrutiny showed important decreases in mean CBF only occurred during rapid orthostasis in some patients. While brain fog symptoms are consistently reported with increasing orthostatic stress, decreased average CBF does not consistently occur and cannot fully account for brain fog in patients with POTS.

Oscillatory Cerebral Blood Flow (OCBF) occurs in POTS and progressively increases during incremental tilt. The blood flow in cerebral arteries is not constant but fluctuates (oscillates) about its mean value. When upright, these oscillations are largely produced by fluctuations in arterial blood pressure at low frequency which capture or "entrain" cerebral blood flow oscillations. Moreover, oscillations in cerebral blood flow and blood pressure are increased, especially in upright POTS patients.

If differences in mean CBF couldn't account for brain fog, perhaps time-dependent changes in CBF could. We reviewed prior upright tilt data and observed prominent oscillatory arterial pressure (OAP) when upright in POTS, which is closely synchronized to OCBF (Figure 1). Oscillations were present in all patients.

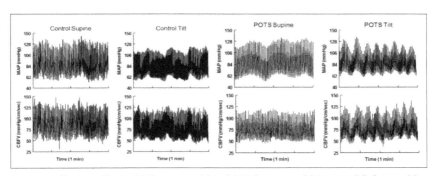

Figure 1: Phasic oscillatory BP (upper panels) and CBF (lower panels) in control (left 4 panels) and POTS patients (right 4 panels) when supine and upright. When upright both BP and CBF became highly oscillatory and synchronous in POTS and to a much lesser degree in control.

We revisited incremental tilt and found monotonically increasing OCBF in POTS patients, but not in controls (Figure 2). Supine, there were predominant slow irregular oscillations of CBF in control and POTS alike, with a frequency range of 0.01 – 0.10 Hz. Oscillatory power was mostly at very low frequencies of 0.01 – 0.03 Hz. When upright, OCBF was concentrated in the 0.07 – 0.12Hz range for POTS. Cerebral blood flow oscillations depend on both blood pressure oscillations and impaired cerebral autoregulation.

This data suggests increased oscillatory cerebral blood flow contributes to postural cognitive deficits in POTS.

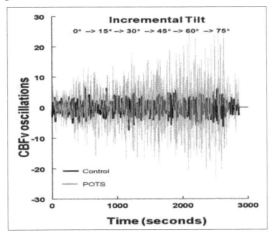

Figure 2 shows increasing OCBF in POTS (gray), compared to control (black) during incremental tilt.

In a recent study1 of 138 POTS patients (88% female), ranging in age from 14 to 29 years, 132 subjects reported brain fog. Subjects were

95

asked to complete a 38-item questionnaire designed to better understand several factors, including triggers and treatments. The most frequently reported brain fog triggers were:

- fatigue (91 %)
- lack of sleep (90 %)
- prolonged standing (87 %)
- dehydration (86 %)
- feeling faint (85 %)

Although aggravated by upright posture, brain fog was reported to persist after assuming a recumbent posture. The most frequently reported interventions for the treatment of brain fog were:

- intravenous saline (77 %)
- stimulant medications (67 %)
- salt tablets (54 %)
- intra-muscular vitamin B-12 injections (48 %)
- midodrine (45 %).

Descriptors for "brain fog" are most consistent with it being a cognitive complaint. Factors other than upright posture may play a role in the persistence of this symptom.

1. Ross AJ, Medow MS, Rowe PC, Stewart JM. What is brain fog? An evaluation of the symptom in postural tachycardia syndrome. Clin Auton Res. 2013;23:305-311.

2. Ocon AJ, Medow MS, Taneja I, Clarke D, Stewart JM. Decreased upright cerebral blood flow and cerebral autoregulation in normocapnic postural tachycardia syndrome. Am J Physiol Heart Circ Physiol. 2009;297:H664-H673.

Dr. Stewart obtained his MD and PhD degrees at the University of Chicago. His internship and residency was in pediatrics at NYU with a fellowship in Pediatric Cardiology at Cornell-New York Hospital. His laboratory funded by the National Institutes of Health for more than 15 years focuses on the study of acute and chronic orthostatic intolerance (OI). He has published widely in the field of autonomic dysfunction and most recently obtained cerebral blood flow correlates of "brain fog" which points towards mechanisms and effective treatment of this disability.

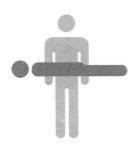

14

ORTHOSTATIC VITALS

Measuring Your Body's Response to Changes in Posture

The orthostatic vitals test is used to evaluate the body's response to a change in position. It examines changes in your heart rate and blood pressure when you are resting, sitting, and standing. Your physician may use this test to get an idea of how your body responds to orthostatic (upright) stress. If you are asked to participate in an orthostatic vitals test it is most helpful to have the test conducted during the morning hours. It is also helpful to wear comfortable, loose fitting clothing because anything that is too tight may cause the results to be inaccurate.

Your physician may also ask you to have a tilt table test, which is a more sophisticated way of measuring orthostatic stress. This test is described in the next chapter.

If you are diagnosed with dysautono-mia, and you have experienced abnormal orthostatic vitals, your doctor may ask you to periodically check your heart rate and/or blood pressure at home. Additionally, when you experience a change in symptoms you may want to check your heart rate and/or blood pressure and share that information with your doctors.

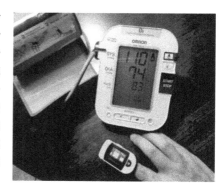

At-home blood pressure cuffs are made either for the arm or the wrist. With a push of a button they record your blood pressure, and some models also show your heart rate. Alternatively, pulse oximeters

14

ORTHOSTATIC VITALS

AN EASY AND MEANINGFUL
INITIAL MEASURE

Physicians and nurse practitioners should consider the orthostatic vitals test in the diagnosis of dysautonomia. This affordable, easy to perform test is a great start in collecting clinical data to go hand in hand with an initial clinical assessment.

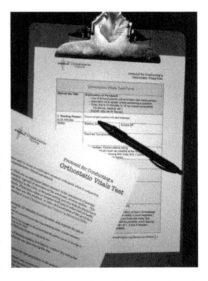

Most practitioners think of orthostatic vitals as having a somewhat limited use (e.g. for the assessment of fluid volume loss in the emergency setting, or orthostatic hypotension in the geriatric population). But, this test, which a nurse or trained staff member can perform in either the clinic or hospital setting, may provide meaningful data about the patient's response to orthostatic stress. More importantly, it may confirm a suspected dysautonomia diagnosis without the use of expensive diagnostic testing.

The use of orthostatic vitals test is recommended in conjunction with a thorough clinical assessment with patients when a dysautonomia diagnosis is suspected. Additionally, physicians may consider using this test when a patient has chronic health problems that have not been successfully managed with typical medications. For example, some patients who have suffered from chronic migraines for years with little

(devices which attach to the end of your finger to monitor both heart rate and the % amount of oxygen that is being distributed through your blood to peripheral (outer) regions of the body) can be purchased at most pharmacies.

If you use at-home instruments such as these, it is important to use them with the understanding of the following cautions:

- At-home monitors can provide false readings and/or inaccurate information. Often these devices are not the same quality as the professional devices used in the hospital or in your physician's office.

- Numbers can be deceiving. The symptoms you experience are more important than the numbers that appear on such devices. If you have any questions, consult your physician.

- If you are asked to collect orthostatic vitals at home by your physician, or for referral to a research program, this is a great time to use at-home devices. However, if you have chronic orthostatic intolerance, it is important to limit the frequency of measuring such data on your own, as it may worsen your symptoms.

Consult your doctor about using at-home diagnostic equipment.

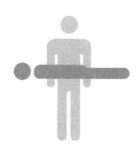

relief from typical migraine medications may under report symptoms of dysautonomia after pain levels are out of control. This behavior is also seen at times in patients with chronic fatigue and fibromyalgia, causing the dysautonomia, which may be the underlying problem, to go undetected.

Requirements for the Orthostatic Vitals Test

The test lasts approximately 15 minutes, is noninvasive, and requires

- A blood pressure cuff,
- Capability to measure the patient's heart rate (e.g., palpating pulse, or pulse oximeter),
- A clock or stopwatch,
- A bed or exam table that is low enough to the ground that the patient can sit on the edge of the table with feet resting on the floor,
- A copy of the Orthostatic Vitals Test Form and instructions (see Appendix B), and
- A quiet room.

Due to the diurnal variability of hemodynamics, it is ideal to conduct this test in the morning hours, but it may be conducted any time during the day. A video demonstration of this procedure is available for viewing at *www.TheDysautonomiaProject.org/Resources/3.*

See the chart on page 103 for abnormal responses in blood pressure and heart rate when standing.

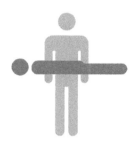

Abnormal Responses in Blood Pressure and Heart Rate when Standing

Often seen in:	Blood Pressure	Heart Rate
Neurogenic Orthostatic Hypotension (NOH)	Consistently drops within 3 minutes of standing by 20 mmHg systolic/ 10mmHg diastolic	Absence of tachycardia
Postural Orthostatic Tachycardia Syndrome (POTS)	*Most cases maintain blood pressure. In some cases a latent drop in blood pressure occurs following tachycardia, as seen in autonomically mediated syncope.*	Increase of 30 bpm (40 bpm in teens) or sustained tachycardia above 120 with symptoms of syncope or presyncope.
Autonomically Mediated Syncope (AMS)*	Drop in blood pressure that leads to syncope or symptoms of presyncope.	*Most cases have little change in heart rate. In some cases the drop in blood pressure occurs following tachycardia as seen in POTS or bradycardia can precede a drop in blood pressure.*

* Also known as neurally mediated, vasovagal and/or neurocardiogenic syncope

An important note

Many variables affect the hemodynamic measures in the orthostatic vitals test, including dehydration, prolonged bed rest, or the common cold and may produce false results. Therefore, the orthostatic vitals test is to be used as a tool to help support a diagnosis of dysautonomia in combination with a comprehensive clinical assessment.

15

THE TILT TABLE TEST

When you walk, exercise, or stand up, the somatic (voluntary) muscles in your legs and abdomen work as a pump to push blood up from the lower part of your body back into the main circulation of your body, including into vital organs such as the heart. Since this interaction can affect your blood pressure and heart rate, an orthostatic vitals test will not produce the most accurate results. However, the tilt table moves your body into an upright position without the use of your muscles, so it does produce more reliable information about how your body reacts to changes in position. Some consider it "the gold standard" of testing for dysautonomias.

Most regional medical centers around the country have tilt table test capabilities, but it is helpful to know that there is wide variation in both procedural protocols and cost. The test is usually performed under the supervision of an electrophysiologist, a cardiologist that specializes in the electrical signals of the heart. Make sure the electrophysiologist who supervises your tilt table test follows updated protocols for administering the test. One way to make sure updated protocols are followed is to share the physician information found in this chapter.

Costs can vary widely between facilities. Usually the medical center charge is between $1,000 and $6,000. If there is more than one location in your area that has the capability of running the test, call the billing offices of all the locations to find out what they charge for the procedure.

The test is fairly easy, and if done properly involves minimal risk. Usually you are asked to rest for a period of time after an IV is inserted. When the resting phase is done, they will take a baseline resting measurement of your blood pressure and heart rate. Then the table slowly moves into an upright position with your feet resting on a small platform. Safety straps, like seatbelts, are used to ensure you do not fall.

15

THE TILT TABLE TEST

Tilt table testing is done to see if standing up (orthostasis) provokes a gradual, progressive fall in blood pressure (orthostatic hypotension), a period of blood pressure instability followed by a sudden fall in blood pressure (neurally mediated hypotension), an excessive increase in pulse rate, as in postural orthostatic tachycardia syndrome (POTS), or autonomically mediated syncope (also known as neurally mediated syncope, neurocardiogenic syncope, or vasovagal syncope).

The testing itself is simple. The patient lies on a stretcher-like table, straps like seat belts are attached around the abdomen and legs, and the patient is tilted upright at an angle. The exact angle used varies from center to center and may be from 60 degrees to 90 degrees. The tilting goes on for up to 45 minutes (this varies from center to center).

If the patient tolerates the tilting for this period, then the patient may receive a drug, such as isoproterenol or nitroglycerine, which may provoke a sudden fall in blood pressure or loss of consciousness.

As soon as the test becomes positive, such as by a sudden fall in blood pressure, the patient is put back into a position lying flat or with the head down. Sometimes fluid is given intravenously. Consciousness rapidly returns once the patient is put back down; however, symptoms such as a sense of imbalance, disorientation, or headache can continue for hours or even days later.

Tilt table testing is a provocative test. The doctors are hoping to reproduce the patient's problem in a controlled laboratory situation.

The testing is quite safe when done by experienced personnel, in a setting where emergency backup is available.

There are some disadvantages of tilt table testing. One is a false-positive test result, especially when a drug is used. In a false-positive test, the results of the test are positive, but some healthy people can have

The test length may vary, but throughout the duration of the test your blood pressure and heart rate are regularly monitored. Should you become symptomatic, have a pronounced drop in blood pressure, or begin to faint, the test should be ended immediately to reduce your risk of fainting.

After the test there is a recovery time. In some autonomic labs IV fluids are also administered. If you have any questions about the test, ask your physician.

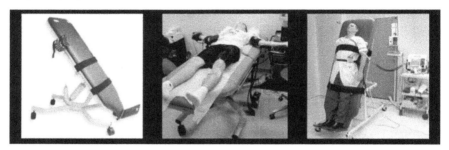

Tilt table testing usually is done with a motorized tilt table.

Tilt table testing is used to evaluate patients with a complaint of fainting or inability to tolerate prolonged standing.

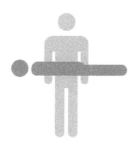

a positive test result, so that a positive test result might not actually mean that anything really is "wrong." More importantly, a false-positive result would lead the doctor to conclude that the condition is fainting, a relatively benign situation, whereas the patient actually has a serious medical problem. This is why a tilt test must be used as a tool in combination with a comprehensive clinical assessment to support a definitive diagnosis.

Another disadvantage is that most tilt table testing does not provide information about disease mechanisms.

"Augmented" tilt table testing involves measurements of physiological functions, such as forearm vascular resistance, and sampling blood for assays of norepinephrine and adrenaline levels. This can be especially helpful for the evaluation of autonomically mediated syncope, as tracking plasma adrenaline and norepinephrine is the only way to detect differential changes in activities of the sympathetic adrenergic and sympathetic noradrenergic systems—sympathoadrenal imbalance—which seems to be a key factor in fainting reactions.

Augmented testing can provide information about mechanisms; however, few centers regularly offer this form of tilt table testing.

If you do not already have access to augmented tilt testing it may be helpful work to add augmented tilt testing at your facility.

Standard tilt table testing is not useful in patients with a persistent fall in blood pressure each time they stand up (orthostatic hypotension), because the results are a foregone conclusion: the blood pressure will fall progressively during the tilting. Augmented tilt table testing, however, can help determine if the orthostatic hypotension results from a form of sympathetic nervous system failure.

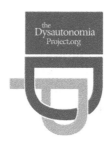

16

LESSONS LEARNED IN TREATING PATIENTS WITH DYSAUTONOMIA

An Interview with Miguel Trevino, MD

By Kelly Freeman

Dr. Miguel Trevino started treating patients with dysautonomia in October 2011. He is in private practice specializing in internal medicine and medication research in Largo, Florida. Although he has no formal training in autonomic medicine, he regularly sees patients with POTS and other forms of dysautonomia. He is also a member of The Dysautonomia Project's Local Medical Advisory Board.

Describe your first patient with dysautonomia.

My first patient was you, Kelly. You came in and had 50 different symptoms, including headache, brain fog, fatigue, dizziness, intestinal issues, palpitations, and jitteriness. You had a ton of symptoms. We went through them all one by one. Your heart rate was going too fast for no reason, so I figured there was something wrong. We ordered a tilt table test, and that's how we got started.

How did you learn about POTS?

I read and learned about POTS on the Internet. As I recall, you directed me to some different websites.

Describe other dysautonomia patients you've recognized and treated.

I have everything from dysautonomia patients that are completely functional to dysautonomia patients that are not functioning at all in their daily lives. In most cases, with trying different treatments, and often a different combination of therapies, you can get them to a place where they are at least more functional than they were. So if their dysfunction was a 10 out of 10 and we can get them to a 4 out of 10, I consider that a great success. A lot of the non-functional patients don't do anything. They don't go out, don't go to the mall, and don't go shopping. Some lie in bed all day. But with a combination of therapies most patients do improve. In some of the really complex cases, I've seen patients that don't improve. Nothing I've tried so far works with them.

Besides POTS, what other forms of dysautonomia have you treated?

I'm not a dysautonomia specialist, so I see a lot of different types of patients on regular basis. For a lot of them who have diabetes, dismotility problems, Parkinson's and other conditions, dysautonomia is also a part of their disease.

Do you think most physicians miss the connection that autonomic dysfunction exists in other conditions?

I think most physicians recognize dysautonomia in general but most don't recognize the variety and amount of symptoms that it can cause. So what I think happens is the patient comes in, has 50 complaints, and they only have 15 minutes to voice them. It's hard to connect that all the symptoms, all 50 of them, are because of dysautonomia. I don't think many physicians make that connection.

Were you familiar with dysautonomia before treating your first patient?

I knew what dysautonomia was, but I didn't know the extent of dysautonomia that people with POTS have.

Do you think dysautonomia is more common than most physicians recognize?

Yes, I do. But I have no statistics on that.

What advice would you give to a physician dealing with a dysautonomia patient for the first time?

When you have somebody with a ton of symptoms, you have to really try to figure out each one of them. And I think an important question is,

"Does it get better when you lie down?" Sometimes the patient doesn't know. But if the symptom generally gets better when the patient lies down, it is probably dysautonomia. There are some symptoms that don't improve when you lie down. And there are a lot of residual effects of epinephrine and norepinephrine when a patient is upright. Once that cascade triggers and tachycardia occurs, the effects can last for days. So one of the most important questions is: "Does it go away when you lie down?"

I'd say in 60% of POTS patients, when you stand them upright, you can see their heart rate go from 80 to 120 in two minutes. So you don't even have to do a 10-minute standing test. As they are standing in front of you, they'll start having symptoms. And the symptoms will go away when you lay them back down. That is a simple thing a doctor could do on a day-to-day basis. This is especially important when you are faced with a patient with so many non-specific symptoms.

What treatment has been most effective in patients you've treated?

It takes three to four months to figure out what is going to work for most patients. It is usually a combination of things that they do along with medications. There is no single treatment that works in every patient. For example, I had a patient with POTS yesterday. The way I found out she had POTS is that she mentioned craving salt since she was a 13- year-old. She is now in her 20s. She gets very sick when she takes beta-blockers, although most patients can tolerate a little bit of beta-blockers. You may have to change treatment and try different ones. There is a great deal of trial and error involved.

Is there anything that is important for physicians and/or patients to know?

The most important thing is to be patient. The biggest problem treating dysautonomia is, it takes time. And nobody has extra time. Time is our most precious commodity.

Miguel Esteban Trevino, MD, is Medical Director of Innovative Research of West Florida, Inc. and maintains a large private internal medicine practice in Clearwater, Florida. 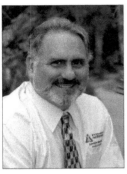 Dr. Trevino has been a Board Certified Internal Medicine Practitioner since 1990. His hospital appointments include both community and private practice in Pinellas County. Innovative Research is at the forefront of Clinical Trial Research, and he has been in charge of over 250 important clinical trials bringing new drugs to market in the United States since 2002. Dr. Miguel Trevino is member of the Tampa Bay Local Medical Advisory Board for The Dysautonomia Project. He has no formal training training in autonomic medicine, but has been treating patients with dysautonomia since 2011.

17

AUTONOMIC CENTERS AND AUTONOMIC FUNCTION TESTING

CONSIDERING FURTHER TESTING?

Physicians in several fields of medicine specialize in dysautonomias. Testing in a specialized autonomic function laboratory may help identify what form of autonomic involvement you have and speed development of an effective therapy program.

You should not feel reluctant to talk to your physician about going to another facility for testing. You will likely find that your physician will actually encourage you to do so because the visit may provide valuable and otherwise unobtainable information that your doctor can use to help you.

> *An educated general practitioner can manage the care of most dysautonomia patients.*

Keep in mind, however, that there are relatively few autonomic function experts and testing laboratories, and an educated general practitioner can take care of most of the management of dysautonomia patients.

As you are deciding whether or not to undergo further diagnostic testing, it is helpful to consider the following:

- **Travel cost and time.** Most insurance companies do not reimburse for your cost to travel to facilities far away. Since insurance plans vary widely, it is important to know if the facility and the doctor you plan to see are covered by your plan.

- **The aim is diagnosis, not necessarily treatment.** Many patients travel to medical centers that are far away for diagnostic testing and return disappointed that they do not

17

AUTONOMIC CENTERS AND AUTONOMIC FUNCTION TESTING

AN OVERVIEW

Once initial assessment is done, depending on the complexity and severity of the case, you may consider referring your patient to an autonomic function clinic at a medical center with expertise in autonomic medicine. There are many diagnostic tests that can be used to evaluate patients with known or suspected dysautonomias. Most centers that perform autonomic function testing use more than one type of test. None use all the tests described.

Tests for dysautonomias can be divided into physiological, neuropharmacologic, neurochemical, neuroimaging, and genetic categories.

Physiological tests involve measurements of a body function in response to a manipulation such as standing, tilt table-testing, or a change in room temperature. There are always several steps between the brain's directing changes in nerve traffic in the autonomic nervous system and the physiological measures that are chosen to track the autonomic changes. Because of this indirectness, results of physiological tests can be difficult to interpret or may not identify a problem accurately.

Neuropharmacologic tests involve giving a drug that affects the autonomic nervous system and measuring its immediate effects, usually on a physiological measure, but sometimes on a biochemical level such as norepinephrine in plasma. Sometimes the results of neuropharmacologic tests can be as difficult to interpret as those of physiologic tests (e.g. when blocking one component of the sympathetic nervous system activates another system compensatorily).

have a new and improved treatment plan or a new doctor who will be following their specific case. Although it varies among facilities, in most cases the physician you visit will make some suggestions about treatments and share them with your local physician to try at some point after you return home.

- **No center has all the diagnostic tests.** It is important to do your research about different autonomic laboratories by looking online at what they offer, and by talking with patients who have experienced care at that location.

- **Know in advance what tests you are scheduled to take.** One of the biggest mistakes patients make is to travel to a town far away for a half-hour consultation with an autonomic specialist who tells them they will have to schedule and return at a future date for certain diagnostic tests. As a patient, it is up to you to research and plan these trips in advance.

- **Plan to stay an extra day or two, just in case.** It is not uncommon, especially in the larger medical centers, for the physician(s) you see to add certain tests or consultations while you are in town. Having an extra day or two planned at the end of your travel may allow you to get more value out of the trip.

The following are tests that are available at many major autonomic laboratories:

Tilt Table Test
Quantitative Sudomotor Axon Reflex Test (QSART)
The Valsalva Maneuver
The Cold Pressor Test
Heart Rate Variability
Blood Volume Testing
Catecholemine Tests
Anitbody Tests
Skin Biopsies

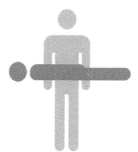

Neurochemical tests involve measuring levels of body chemicals, such as the catecholamines, norepinephrine, and epinephrine, either under resting conditions or in response to physiological or neuropharmacologic manipulations. Several factors influence plasma norepinephrine levels, besides release from sympathetic nerves, so these tests also can be difficult to interpret. Neurochemical tests can be done on blood samples that are drawn while the patient is at rest lying down, or during a physiological manipulation such as exercise, or during tilting on a tilt table, or during a neuropharmacologic manipulation. Relatively few centers have a clinical neurochemistry laboratory to carry out the assays. The results can be affected significantly by dietary constituents, drugs, or dietary supplements the patient is taking and by the exact conditions at the time of sampling. There is no chemical test of parasympathetic nervous system activity. This is because an enzyme breaks down acetylcholine, the main chemical messenger of the parasympathetic nervous system, almost as soon as acetylcholine enters body fluids such as the plasma.

Neuroimaging tests involve actually visualizing parts of the autonomic nervous system, such as the sympathetic nerves in the heart. Neuroimaging tests, involve actually visualizing the autonomic nerve supply in body organs. As yet there is no accepted neuroimaging test to visualize parasympathetic nerves. Cardiac MIBG SPECT neuroimaging is widely available in most academic centers. Sympathetic neuroimaging via PET imaging is done in few centers, and although this type of testing can produce striking images of the sympathetic innervation of the heart, this provides mainly anatomic information about whether sympathetic nerves are present. It is still unclear whether sympathetic neuroimaging can provide information about whether or not those nerves are functioning normally. Neuroimaging can also be used to identify brain diseases that are associated with dysautonomias. For instance, different types of scans can identify the loss of nerve terminals that contain dopamine in the brain in Parkinson's disease, or identify abnormalities of brain structures that regulate the autonomic nervous system.

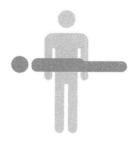

End of Patient section.

Genetic tests involve analyses of genetic material (DNA) for abnormalities of specific genes that produce or predispose to the development of particular diseases.

Which Test Are Done Where?

Few centers conduct comprehensive autonomic function testing. Physiological tests, such as measurements of heart rate responses to the Valsalva maneuver, are readily available. Neuropharmacologic tests, such as the QSART and skin biopsies, are done in several specialized autonomic function testing centers. Neurochemical tests, such as plasma norepinephrine and adrenaline levels, are done in fewer centers. And as of this writing, neuroimaging tests are rarely available in the United States because third party payers don't cover them. At this point, there are only a few genetic tests for particular forms of dysautonomia, such as familial dysautonomia.

At a minimum the battery of autonomic function tests at a given medical center should be able to identify abnormalities of regulation of the circulation by the sympathetic noradrenergic system, sweating by the sympathetic cholinergic system, and heart rate by the parasympathetic nervous system.

Other types of testing would depend on the particular problem the patient is facing. For instance, assessment of dysautonomia in a patient with evidence of a neurodegenerative disease such as Parkinson's disease, may be complimented with neuroimaging to examine both dopamine centers in the brain and the supply of sympathetic nerves in the heart; while for assessment of postural tachycardia syndrome, measurement of blood volume may be indicated.

Overview of Autonomic Function Tests

Note: The list on the next two pages is an overview. For a more complete list of autonomic function tests, see Principles of Autonomic Medicine available at www.TheDysautonomiaProject/resources/2.

The asterisked tests below (*), or variations of these tests, are used at many autonomic laboratories along with tilt table testing. Check with the lab to ensure the indicated test is available.

Overview of Autonomic Function Tests

PHYSIOLOGICAL TESTS

The Valsalva Maneuver *	One of the most important clinical physiological tests for autonomic failure. The maneuver consists of blowing against a resistance for several seconds and then relaxing. Beat to beat blood pressure monitoring is required. Valuable for diagnosing sympathetic neurocirculatory failure, but is of no value in differential diagnosis among autonomic failure syndromes. (See figures 1 & 2)
Thermoregulatory Sweat Test	Examines sympathetic cholinergic nervous system function from the sweating response to external heat. Perspiration is visualized by sprinkling all over the body indicator powder, which turns color when wetted. Can detect small fiber neuropathy, sympathetic cholinergic denervation in the feet or hands, or denervation in large areas of the trunk.
Heart Rate Variability *	Measures the inter-beat heart rate using analysis of heart rate variability in a time domain. Normal variability appears like a bell shaped curve, getting wider with increased variability. In many forms of heart disease, such as CHF, and in most forms of chronic autonomic failure, the heart rate becomes more stable, narrowing the bell-shaped curve.
Ambulatory Blood Pressure Monitoring	Blood pressure is monitored at predetermined times through daily activities and sleeping to assess patterns in BP variation.
The Cold Pressor Test *	Blood pressure is monitored when the patient dunks a hand into a container of ice-cold water and keeps the hand immersed. This rapidly increases the blood pressure by increasing activity of the sympathetic noradrenergic system.

NEUROPHARMACOLOGICAL TESTS

Quantitative Sudomotor Axon Reflex Test (QSART) *	The QSART tests the ability of sympathetic nerves in the skin to release acetylcholine and increase sweat production in a small capsule placed on the skin. (Usually a lower limb.)
Skin Biopsies*	Usually skin biopsy samples contain tiny blood vessels. The walls of arterioles receive sympathetic noradrenergic nerve fibers, which can be identified by dopamine-beta-hydroxylase (DBH) or tyrosine hydroxylase (TH) staining. Especially useful in evaluation of small fiber neuropathies.
Clonidine Suppression Testing	Clonidine decreases release of norepinephrine from sympathetic nerves and decreases blood pressure by stimulating alpha-2 adrenoceptors in the brain, in blood vessel walls, and on sympathetic nerve terminals. Used mainly to evaluate pheochromocytoma or hypernoreadrenergic hypertension, this test is based on effects of the drug on blood pressure and on plasma levels of norepinephrine.

NEUROCHEMICAL/BIOCHEMICAL TESTS	
Blood Volume *	In the blood volume test, blood volume is calculated from the concentration and amount of a drug in the bloodstream using a radioactive tag, measurements over time, and algebra to calculate total blood volume. This test is especially useful in determining hypovolemia in chronic orthostatic intolerance.
Catecholemine Tests *	**Plasma Norepinephrine (NE)** NE is the main chemical messenger of the sympathetic noradrenergic system, which doctors have often used as an index of sympathetic nervous system "activity" in the body as a whole. Supine plasma NE levels normally range from about 100 to about 500 pg/mL and double upon standing. **Plasma Epinephrine (EPI)** Compared to the plasma norepinephrine level, which is complexly and indirectly related to sympathetic noradrenergic system "activity" in the body as a whole, the plasma epinephrine (adrenaline) level is a fairly direct indicator of activity of the sympathetic adrenergic system (adrenomedullary hormonal system). Plasma adrenaline (epinephrine) is used to test the sympathetic adrenergic system (SAS).
Antibody Tests *	One mechanism by which autonomic nerves could be harmed is by auto-immunity, as organisms express proteins that are expressed in the autonomic nervous system. The immune system raises an antibody to that protein, which damages or interferes with the function of the nerves. Probably the most well characterized form of auto-immune attack is autoimmune autonomic neuropathy from a circulating antibody to the neuronal nicotinic receptor. In autoimmune autonomic ganglionopathy (AAG), the attack is sufficiently severe and generalized to cause all components of the autonomic nervous system to fail. Cancer cells can produce antibodies to proteins expressed by autonomic nerves ("paraneoplastic syndrome"). Anti-Hu antibodies (also known as Type 1 anti-neuronal nuclear antibody, ANNA-1) are especially common in small cell lung cancers.
NEUROIMAGING TESTS	
Cardiac Sympathetic Neuroimaging via PET scan	Using PET scan and radioactive markers, it shows sympathetic nerves in the heart travel with the coronary arteries. Because neuroimaging tests have limited resolution, the imaging does not show individual nerves but gives a general picture, and since the nerves are found throughout the heart muscle, the picture looks very much like a scan of the heart muscle. (Very limited access in the US today.)
Cardiac MIBG SPECT Imaging	Involves visualization of sympathetic noradrenergic innervation of the left ventricle myocardium. While these images are not as clean and quantitative as PET imaging they are widely available at most academic centers.
GENETIC TESTS	Several genetic tests are available for specific dysautonomias, including familial dysautonomia, DBH deficiency, NET deficiency, and Menkes disease.

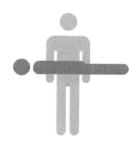

Figure 1

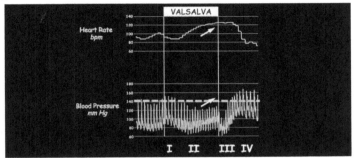

Normal blood pressure (BP) and heart rate (HR) responses during the 4 phases of the Valsalva maneuver. Beat to beat blood pressure monitoring is used.

Figure 2

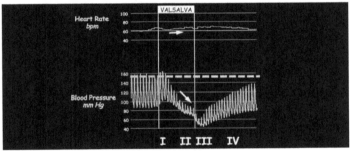

Abnormal blood pressure (BP) and heart rate (HR) responses to the Valsalva maneuver, indicating failure to regulate the sympathetic and parasympathetic nervous systems correctly.

18

COEXISTING CONDITIONS

For most dysautonomia patients there are so many symptoms to discuss during a doctor's appointment that it is easy to miss discussing important symptoms that may give your doctor insight about an underlying cause or coexisting condition. Here is a table of common complaints associated with various conditions. If you have experienced these symptoms, discuss them with your physician while keeping in mind that there could be other causes of these symptoms. They may be signs of coexisting conditions.

Common Coexisting Conditions List

Condition	Symptoms Sometime Seen
Auto-Immunity	Dry eyes, dry mouth, dilated pupils, joint pain, swollen lymph nodes.
Chronic Regional Pain Syndrome	Constant burning pain, pain that is disproportionate (more than what it should be), one limb that is or has experienced pain and swelling with or without trauma.
Diabetes	Chronic pain in feet, urinary problems, erectile problems in males
Ehlers-Danlos Syndrome	Hypermobile joints, history of multiple dislocated joints, stretchy skin, very thin skin
Mast Cell Activation Syndrome	Flushing (dry, hot, red face or upper body), multiple hypersensitivities, hives, anaphylaxis
Sleep Disorders	Difficulty staying awake, difficulty sleeping, commonly experience unrefreshed sleep.
Small Fiber Neuropathy	Pins and needles, burning and/or numb sensations of extremities, especially at rest.

* This list includes the most common conditions and is not intended to be exhaustive. It may change based on feedback of The Dysautonomia Project members and advisors. Check our website for the most updated list at: www.TheDysautonomiaProject.org/Resources/4.

18

COEXISTING CONDITIONS

Evaluation of Coexisting Conditions

Dysautonomias can occur as a primary condition, as in pure autonomic failure, or as a condition secondary to another where, in most cases, the dysautonomia is a compensatory reaction to something else going on in the body, as seen in paraneoplastic syndromes. It can also occur as coexisting condition, as seen in "The Triple Threat" of POTS, Ehlers-Danlos Syndrome, and mast cell activation disorders.

Diabetes

Dysautonomia is common in diabetes, and is associated with worse outcomes. Although peripheral neuropathy is well known in diabetes, the understanding of the autonomic dysfunction and/or failure is not well known.

Diabetes is probably the most common cause of autonomic neuropathy. Among patients with diabetes, the occurrence of autonomic neuropathy is an adverse prognostic factor. Diabetes often involves chronic pain in the feet (painful diabetic neuropathy). Loss of sympathetic noradrenergic innervation in the feet accompanies the neuropathy.

Diabetics can also have neurogenic orthostatic hypotension, with evidence of failure of baroreflex regulation of sympathetic noradrenergic system outflows. Poor control of the urinary bladder, erectile dysfunction, resting tachycardia, diarrhea and other GI symptoms may also suggest a coexisting diabetic autonomic neuropathy.

The following five chapters, along with Chapter 34, by contributing authors cover some of the more common coexisting, as well as specific conditions, of dysautonomia.

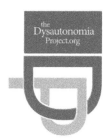

19

SMALL FIBER NEUROPATHY

by Kamal R. Chémali, MD

The term "small fiber neuropathy" may not be familiar to a lot of patients with a disorder of the autonomic nervous system, but the concept of involvement of the "small fibers" in many of these disorders is of the utmost importance.

The "small fibers," as opposed to the "large fibers," refers to the thinnest, unmyelinated (bare axons) or thinly-myelinated nerves of the peripheral nervous system, which we also call C-fibers and A-delta fibers, respectively. These nerves mainly are known to mediate the so-called "protopathic sensory modalities," i.e., the perception of pain and temperature. Their initial dysfunction (which we could consider as a state of suffering of the nerves) leads to over-firing and results in a sensation of burning and/or pins and needles or sharp stabbing pain, predominantly in the distal extremities such as the feet or hands, and typically occurs at rest or at night. Because the small fibers are present throughout the body, these abnormal sensations can also, in rarer instances, be present in other areas of the body, such as the face, the tip of the nose, the perineal region, etc. We call these "positive symptoms." On the other hand, when the pathological process becomes more advanced, these nerves may degenerate and die, leading to "negative symptoms," mainly numbness. When the two phenomena occur simultaneously, it is not uncommon for patients to describe their symptoms paradoxically, as "painful numbness."

Patients often disregard these symptoms, either because they are mild and do not interfere with their daily life, or because, if they have diabetes, for example, they are told that "burning feet" are a normal manifestation of this disease. When patients with small fiber neuropathy start seeking medical attention, the pain or discomfort is generally severe enough to affect their sleep, their ability to walk, exercise, etc.

In mild or severe cases, and even in sub-clinical cases, neurologists are often able to detect the presence of a small fiber neuropathy during the neurological examination by documenting decreased sensation to pinprick, cold or heat, and sometimes vibration, worse distally and improving proximally (a phenomenon called "sensory gradient" or "length-dependent").

Why is a small-fiber neuropathy important in the dysautonomias? Because the unmyelinated C-fibers also mediate autonomic functions and form a large majority of the peripheral autonomic nervous system. Indeed, we think that there are 2 different populations of small-fibers: the ones that mediate somatic functions, and those that are responsible for autonomic functions. The former population of fibers is studied using laboratory tests, such as the "Quantitative Sensory Testing" (QST) or a skin biopsy. The latter group is studied using autonomic function tests, particularly "sudomotor" tests (sweat tests), such as the Quantitative Sudomotor Axon Reflex Test (QSART) or the Thermoregulatory Sweat Test (TST).

Detecting an abnormality in somatic, autonomic small-fiber function, or both, in patients with symptoms attributable to the autonomic nervous system raises the diagnosis of "autonomic small-fiber neuropathy," which, in turn, opens the door to a list of potential underlying causes of the dysautonomia, which the physician needs to look for in detail. Some of these causes could be controllable, and possibly reversible in certain instances. Treating the underlying cause, if found, as opposed to treating symptoms only, increases the chances of improving the dysautonomia in some patients.

Dr. Chémali is a specialist of neurology at Sentara Medical Group in Norfolk, VA. He earned his medical degree from the Lebanese University Faculty of Medical Sciences. He completed internships at Lebanese University Faculty of Medical Sciences and at Staten Island University Hospital, and his neurology residency at University

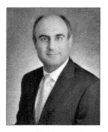 *Hospitals of Cleveland and Case Western Reserve University. He then completed fellowship training in Clinical Neurophysiology, Electromyography and Neuromuscular Diseases at Cleveland Clinic. Dr. Chémali is certified by the American Board of Psychiatry and Neurology and by the American Board of Electrodiagnostic Medicine. Among his many leadership roles and professional affiliations, Dr. Chémali is a member of the American Academy of Neurology, where he serves as a course director; the American Association of Neuromuscular and Electrodi-diagnostic Medicine; and the American Autonomic Section of the American Academy of Neurology. He has a special interest in Music Medicine and Neurological Music Therapy.*

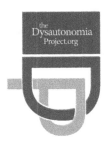

20

AUTOIMMUNITY AND DYSAUTONOMIA

by Steven Vernino, MD, PhD

There is an association between autoimmune conditions and dysautonomia. Both autoimmunity and dysautonomia are common and occur more often in females than in males. Both are challenging to diagnose and manage because of diverse clinical presentations. There are some instances of autonomic disorders that are directly cases by autoimmunity (the immune system directly interacting with the autonomic nerves). In many other cases, dysautonomia may be the secondary consequence of a chronic systemic autoimmune illness causing deconditioning and release of inflammatory mediators throughout the body. Although autoimmune dysautonomia exists, our ability to easily recognize it is lacking even using sophisticated autonomic assessments and antibody testing.

The immune system is critically important for survival, as it constantly surveys for infection (e.g., bacteria, viruses), cancer cells, and other foreign material (e.g., toxins, venom). The immune system can specifically kill pathogens or cancer cells and also clean up damaged tissues after injury. A healthy immune system provides continuous monitoring of both foreign and internal dangers throughout the body, while ignoring or tolerating normal healthy tissue.

In autoimmune disorders the immune system inappropriately attacks normal parts of the body, including joints, skin, gut, blood vessels, muscles, nerves, and internal organs. In the case of infected, damaged or precancerous cells, autoimmunity can be helpful, but autoimmune disease occurs when attack on normal tissues occurs spontaneously or persists after a threat is gone. Autoimmunity can occur spontaneously, particularly in patients with a strong family history of autoimmune disease, or it can develop in the context of a stressful stimulus to the body, such as surgery, viral infection, or cancer.

Autoimmunity can include the production of antibodies that react with targets in healthy cells, the excessive release of inflammatory mediators (such as histamine and interleukin proteins), or activation of immune cells attacking normal tissue. In some cases, the immune system directly targets parts of the autonomic nervous system. The following table provides an overview of several autoimmune conditions associated with autonomic problems (see table next page).

In cases where an autoimmune condition is known, it is not uncommon to overlook the coexisting dysautonomia which may be improved with treatments such as those listed under the treatments section in this book, including volume expansion and exercise, among others. In cases where the dysautonomia is known, it may be helpful to consider if a coexisting underlying autoimmune disorder is present. In such cases, it may be very difficult to effectively manage the symptoms of the dysautonomia unless the autoimmune condition is identified and treated.

When investigating patients with dysautonomia, it is helpful to conduct a detailed history that addresses multiple organ symptoms. The rapid onset of symptoms after a prodromal illness may suggest an immune-mediated condition. The presence of skin rash or swollen salivary glands can point to particular disorders. Autonomic testing and nerve conduction studies can be used to identify the presence of neuropathy and to characterize the type of autonomic dysfunction. Patients with objective evidence of autonomic neuropathy are more likely to have an underlying cause found compared to those with dysautonomia but intact autonomic nerves. Laboratory testing, including antibody tests, may be helpful in identifying an underlying autoimmune condition but, unfortunately, many serological markers are not completely sensitive or specific. It is important to understand that ancillary tests alone are often insufficient for a proper diagnosis. Therefore, a good appreciation of the complex interaction between the immune system and autonomic function is essential.

Autoimmune Conditions Associated with Dysautonomia

(This table is a sample list and is not intended to be exhaustive.)

Autoimmune Condition	Immune System Typically Attacks	Typical Autonomic Signs or Symptoms	Other features
Autoimmune Autonomic Ganglionopathy (AAG)	Neurons in autonomia ganglia	Orthostatic hypotension (OH), gastrointestinal issues, urinary retention	Ganglionic AChR antibodies in 50% of patients
Paraneoplastic autonomic neuropathy	Autonomic nerves and neurons	Gastroparesis, orthostatic hypotension	Association with small cell lung cancer (anti-Hu antibodies)
Autoimmune Encephalopathy	Central nervous system	Excessive sweating, labile blood pressure and heart rate	Antibodies against VGKC* or NMDA receptors
Guillain-Barré syndrome	Peripheral nervous system	Labile blood pressure and heart rate, constipation.	Autonomic neuropathy
Sjogrens syndrome	Moisture-secreting glands of eyes and mouth	Dry eyes and dry mouth, fatigue, orthostatic tachycardia	SSA/SSB antibodies.
Celiac Disease	Gluten proteins and the small bowel	Gastrointestinal issues	Peripheral neuropathy or ataxia
Systemic Lupus Erythematosus (SLE)	Tissues throughout the body	Skin rashes, parastheseias, fatigue	Peripheral neuropathy

* VGKC = voltage-gated potassium channel complex

Dr. Vernino is Professor and Academic Vice-Chair in the Department of Neurology & Neurotherapeutics at the University of Texas Southwestern Medical Center in Dallas. He also holds the Dr. Bob and Jean Smith Foundation Distinguished Chair in Neuromuscular Disease Research. Dr. Vernino is the director of the clinical autonomic

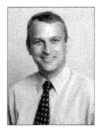 *laboratory and clinic at UT Southwestern. He has been involved with research related to autonomic disorders for the past 20 years. His major contribution to the field was the discovery of ganglionic AChR antibodies and the role of these antibodies as a cause for autonomic failure (autoimmune autonomic ganglionopathy). He has also contributed to research studies aimed at the treatment of autonomic disorders and autoimmune neurological disorders such as paraneoplastic syndromes and autoimmune encephalitis.*

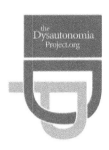

2 1

THE TRIPLE THREAT

POTS, MCAD & Connective
Tissue Disorders

by Lisa Klimas, MS

Dysautonomia refers to a group of symptoms that suggests poor control of the autonomic nervous system (ANS). Diminished action of involuntary control mechanisms results in a number of symptoms, including exercise intolerance, shortness of breath, excessive fatigue, and heart rate and blood pressure disturbances. A number of conditions are marked by autonomic dysfunction, including postural orthostatic tachycardia syndrome (POTS) and orthostatic intolerance (OI), among others. Dysautonomia is thought to affect over 70 million people worldwide.

Dysautonomia can occur secondarily to a number of other conditions. Associations have been made between autonomic dysfunction and heritable connective tissue disorders, including Ehlers Danlos Syndrome (EDS). These disorders are associated with a wide array of clinical manifestations and range from superficial to life-threatening. Most heritable connective tissue disorders are associated with known mutations, though some have no known associated mutation, as in hypermobility type EDS (HEDS).[1]

HEDS patients often suffer recurrent joint dislocations and chronic pain, but the symptoms most frequently linked to impairment and poor quality of life involve other systems. Symptoms can include syncope, palpitations, diarrhea, constipation, severe fatigue, and orthostatic intolerance. These can be triggered or worsened by standing upright, physical exercise, consumption of large meals, and exposure to heat, including hot water. Fatigue is the second most common patient complaint in HEDS, following pain.

One study found that in one cohort with HEDS, 74% of the patients had orthostatic intolerance, with POTS the most common form (41%). HEDS was associated with increased sympathetic activity while resting, including higher heart rate. Sympathetic compensation was diminished in response to cardiovascular challenge, such as tilt table tests and Valsalva maneuvers.[2]

Degree of skin extensibility was a significant predictor for severity of dysautonomia. Higher levels of pain were associated with increased heart rate during rest and testing. Findings point to insufficient vasoconstriction by sympathetic nerves.[3] Peripheral neuropathy has been offered by multiple researchers as the link between dysautonomia and heritable connective tissue disorders, but evidence is not yet available to support this suspicion.

The association of mast cell activation disease (MCAD) with EDS and dysautonomia has emerged over time. Mast cell activation disease (MCAD) is marked by allergic-type reactions in response to a variety of triggers, including foods, physical and emotional stress, temperature extremes, fragrances, vibration, and sunlight, among many others. These reactions primarily occur independently of IgE signaling. Common symptoms include flushing, hives, itching, GI symptoms, and sleep disturbances. MCAD patients can experience severe anaphylaxis to seemingly inert stimuli that causes them to require aggressive management, including epinephrine. [4]

MCAD may be proliferative (systemic mastocytosis, SM) or not (mast cell activation syndrome, MCAS). MCAS offers a similar clinical experience without elevation of the most well-known SM marker, tryptase. Diagnosis often relies upon use of 24-hour urine tests for n-methylhistamine and D2 or 9a, 11b-F2 prostaglandin.

MCAD is marked by release of mast cell mediators, including vasoactive moieties, including histamine.[5] A 2006 paper reported the co-occurrence of mast cell activation in some POTS patients, as determined by urinary methylhistamine level $\geq$ 230 µg/g creatinine associated with a flushing episode. The population of interest in this study also demonstrated an increased heart rate of ≥ 30 mm Hg within five minutes of standing, as opposed to the more commonly observed orthostatic hypotension or gradual decrease in heart rate more often seen in patients with neurogenic POTS.[6]

The most common presentation of these co-occurring conditions is MCAS/HEDS/POTS. A recent communication found that in a cohort of 15 POTS/hypermobility patients, 66% of patients with verified POTS and EDS were positive for symptoms of a mast cell disorder.[6] This triple threat of dysautonomia, heritable connective tissue disorder, and mast cell activation disease can result in disability and poor quality of life for patients.

[1] De Wandele, I. et al. Dysautonomia and its underlying mechanisms in the hypermobility type of Ehlers-Danlos syndrome. Seminars in Arthritis and Rheumatism 44 (2014) 93-100.

[2] Gazit J. et al. Dysautonomia in the joint hypermobility syndrome. Am J Med. 2003 Jul; 115(1) :33-40.

[3] De Paepe, A., Malfair, F., 2012. The Ehlers-Danlos syndrome, a disorder with many faces. Clin Genet. 82, 1-11.

[4] Molderings GJ et al. Mast cell activation disease: a concise practical guide for diagnostic workup and therapeutic options. J Hematol Oncol 2011; 4:10.

[5] Shibao C. et al. Hyperadrenergic postural tachycardia syndrome in mast cell activation disorders. Hypertension 2005; 45:385-390.

[6] Cheung I, Vadas P. A new disease cluster: mast cell activation syndrome, postural orthostatic tachycardia sundrome, and Ehlers-Danlos syndrome. 2015 Feb; 135(2, Supplement): AB65.

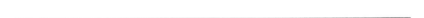

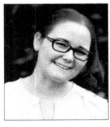

Lisa Klimas is a Senior Scientist at the Novartis Institute for Biomedical Research with expertise in both microbiology and molecular biology. With a focus on diagnostics development, she currently develops companion diagnostics for clinical trial drugs for both oncology and rare diseases. With microbiology expertise in infectious diseases, she has co-authored two papers on the use of FISH assays for diagnosing bloodstream infections. She received her BS in Biological Sciences and MS in in Biology from the University of Massachusetts and has been working in research and development environments for many years. She is a strong believer that cur-

rent, accurate health related information should be easily accessible to anyone who wants it, especially in rare disease communities. When she's not writing about mast cell disease and related conditions, she is talking fast, listening to punk music, doing yoga, hanging out with her dogs, avoiding undercooked egg whites and direct sunlight, and living a pretty great life with multiple chronic diseases. You can find more of her writing at www.mastattack.org.

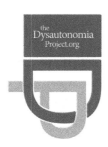

22

MAST CELL ACTIVATION SYNDROME

A Chameleon that Confounds Diagnostics and Treatment for Other Diseases

by Lawrence B. Afrin, MD

Mast Cell Activation Syndrome (MCAS) is the most common form of systemic mast cell disease and appears to underlie symptoms experienced by patients with varying forms of dysautonomia. Only recently have experts identified this condition. It can now be diagnosed with a clinical exam, including a detailed medical history and laboratory tests to confirm the presence of abnormal mast cell activation.

Among other functions, mast cells help protect the body from harmful environmental stimuli by releasing, when activated, specific chemical mediators, including histamine, leukotrienes, prostaglandins, and other inflammatory cytokines. Mast cells are found in every tissue throughout the body and contain an estimated 60-200 different chemical mediators. Like systemic mastocytosis, which additionally features proliferation of mast cells in the bone marrow, MCAS patients present with focal and systemic symptoms due to the abnormal release of inflammatory cytokines by degranulation or exocytosis. When mast cells are activated, they often cause a cascade of symptoms that affect many, perhaps even all, organ systems, including circulatory, neurologic, digestive, etc., with symptoms as innocuous as a skin rash or as life-threatening as anaphylaxis. Mast cells can be activated spontaneously or triggered by various chemical, sensory, or emotional stimuli. The exact set of symptoms varies greatly from patient to patient, appearing a bit like a chameleon upon presentation and often confounding diagnostic testing and treatments of other diseases.

For instance, inflammatory mediators of mast cells can play an auxiliary role in autoimmune diseases, can cause an unusual form of myocardial infarction known as Kounis syndrome, and can appear as cyclical anaphylactic and/or anaphylactoid circulatory shock, to name just a few widely heterogeneous presentations. The trademark similarity between all patients with MCAS is the presence of multiple unexplained symptoms (usually inflammatory ± allergic) in many, if not all, organ systems (though that finding by itself is not diagnostic).

Early research on the epidemiology of MCAS suggests that as many as 14-17% of the general population may be affected (Haenisch, B, et al., Immunology 2012;137:197-205; Molderings, GJ, et al., PLoS One 2013;8(9):e76241). Because MCAS has only been recognized recently and there is a general lack of awareness of it within the medical community, most MCAS patients today remain undiagnosed. And, due to the non-specific nature of almost every symptom of the disease, the diagnosis virtually always goes unsuspected.

When a patient with an already definitively diagnosed ailment—particularly a patient with chronic multisystem polymorbidity, generally of an inflammatory theme—presents for evaluation, it is important for the physician to consider whether or not the presenting symptoms are typical for the definitively diagnosed ailment. If not, it is important to consider the possibility that a co-morbid (and potentially underlying/unifying) illness may be present. Additionally, the severity of MCAS often permanently "steps up" to a higher baseline level following severe physical or psychological stress.

How is Mast Cell Activation Syndrome (MCAS) diagnosed?

1. **Establish suspicion of the disease.** Are there classic signs of mast cell activation (e.g., unprovoked flushing or anaphylaxis)? Are there symptoms of mast cell activation in many, if not all organ systems? (See table of systemic findings.) Are there more symptoms or signs than can be explained by the patient's existing, definitively established diagnoses? Are there "odd" symptoms and findings?

2. **Laboratory testing.** If there are skin lesions suggestive of the cutaneous forms of mastocytosis, they should be biopsied to look for that disease. Also, the serum tryptase level remains a good "fork in the road." If it's persistently above the 20 ng/ml cut-off defined as one of the WHO criteria for systemic mastocytosis (SM), then further evaluation should be directed toward SM. If not, further evaluation should be directed toward additional mast cell mediator testing in blood or urine samples, including elevations in specific and/or non-specific metabolites such as histamine (or its breakdown products), heparin, chromogranin A, prostaglandin D2, or leukotriene E4. A review published in 2014 in the World Journal of Hematology goes on to discuss the details and nuances of properly performing all of this testing, and it's freely available at *http://www.wjgnet.com/2218-6204/pdf/v3/i1/1.pdf*. It should be noted that without wide awareness of the diagnostic criteria for MCAS within the medical community, physicians with knowledge of systemic mastocytosis may mistakenly test solely for serum tryptase, which is commonly elevated in systemic mastocytosis, yet in most cases is within normal limits in MCAS patients.

3. **Additionally,** a positive response to mast cell activation treatments (e.g. therapeutic doses of H1 & H2 antihistamines, aspirin, corticosteroids, among many others) directed at controlling mast cells or blocking the effects of released mast cell mediators, is a significant finding to support the diagnosis but is not required, as finding effective, let alone optimal, treatment often requires patience and persistence through trials of many therapies as no predictors of effective therapy have yet been identified.

There is currently no cure for MCAS, but most patients eventually find treatment that helps bring improvement in symptoms. Although a long list of pharmacological and non-pharmacological treatment options have been found to be helpful in improving symptoms, due to the wide variation in biochemistries between patients along with the heterogeneity of symptoms, a great deal of trial and error is often required before a significant improvement in symptoms is achieved. It should be noted that treatments commonly found helpful in initially diagnosed conditions might worsen symptoms in patients with MCAS. For instance, low dose beta blockers, known to be helpful in improving symptoms including tachycardia for most patients, are also well documented as worsening symptoms in patients with both POTS and MCAS and potentially even blocking the lifesaving effect of epinephrine when trying to treat anaphylaxis.

Systemic mast cell disease was once thought to be just the fairly rare case of cutaneous or systemic mastocytosis, but due to findings in recent years MCAS is now known to be more common. Patients with a wide assortment of symptoms in multiple or all organ systems (including idiopathic dysautonomia, irritable bowel syndrome, interstitial cystitis, idiopathic anaphylaxis, and some subsets of fibromyalgia, etc.) that are not explained by some other condition should consider MCAS as a possible underlying diagnosis.

Systemic Findings in MCAS	
Multi-System	Fatigue, malaise, pain, and inflammation.
Integumentary	Flushing, Trouble with skin, hair, nails, and teeth. All manners of rash and skin lesions, including hives, urticaria pigmentosa (UP), and others.
Ocular/Ophthalmologic	Waxing and waning inflammation of the conjunctival tissue, often described as burning, sandy, dry or gritty; difficulty focusing; blepharospasm (trembling of the eyelid); visual disturbances; pupilomotor dysfunction.
Otologic	Tinnitus, ear pain, hearing loss, and ear drum spasms.
Sinonasal	Congestion and frequent infections.
Oral/Pharyngeal	Mouth sores, sore throat, and difficulty swallowing.
Lymphatic	Swollen lymph nodes and enlarged spleen.
Pulmonary	Shortness of breath, bronchial constriction, and dyspnea.
Cardiovascular	Non-cardiac chest pain, palpitations, tachycardia, hypertension, hypotension, syncope, POTS, arrhythmias, and Kounis Syndrome (allergic angina).
Gastrointestinal	Abdominal pain, diarrhea, constipation, nausea, IBS, gastroparesis.

Neurological	Memory and word finding difficulties, headache, neuropathic pain, difficulty in concentrating.
Urinary and Genitourinary	Urinary Tract Infections and Interstitial Cystitis.
Musculoskeletal and Joint	Muscle, joint or bone pain.
Neuropsychiatric	Anxiety, depression, sleeplessness.
Endocrinologic/Metabolic	Wide array of abnormal hormonal and metabolic laboratory results, especially common ferritin and magnesium levels and brittle bones.
Hematologic	Coagulation, easy bruising.
Immunologic	Infections and environmental hypersensitivies, autoimmunities and cancers

---

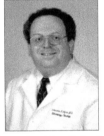

Dr. Afrin is an Associate Professor of Medicine, Hematology, Oncology & Transplantation at the University of Minnesota. He earned a B.S. in Computer Science at Clemson University in 1984 and then an MD at the Medical University of South Carolina (MUSC) in 1988, where he also pursued an internal medicine residency and hematology/oncology clinical and re-search fellowships. While on faculty at MUSC 1995-2014, he was active in undergraduate and graduate medical education, educational and IT administration, and practice and research in hematology/oncology and medical informatics. Since the mid-2000s, his clinical work has increasingly focused in hematology, especially mast cell disease; he also directed MUSC's myeloproliferative neoplasms clinical trials program. He joined the University of Minnesota in 2014. He has served on national panels on oncology edu-cation and quality care, and speaks widely in his areas of focus. He has an extensive record of peer-reviewed publications, and serves on the editorial boards for several journals and on the Medical Advisory Board for The Mastocytosis Society.

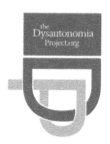

23

SLEEP DISORDERS IN THE DYSAUTONOMIAS

by Alan Pocinki, MD, FACP

Non-restorative sleep is a common feature of the dysautonomias and conditions associated with autonomic dysfunction, such as Ehlers-Danlos and chronic fatigue syndrome (CFS). In my experience, sleep studies in these patients often show frequent disruptions and/or reduced deep sleep; and treatments that are successful in reducing arousals and increasing deep sleep yield symptomatic improvements in the quality of sleep.

Disruptions in the continuity of sleep are termed either awakenings (defined as lasting longer than 30 seconds, though most people will not recall being awake unless they have been awake for at least 2 minutes) or arousals, if less than 30 seconds long. Arousals are usually termed either respiratory, if related to respiratory difficulty such as apnea; movement related, as in periodic limb movements of sleep; or, if neither of these causes is apparent, "spontaneous." Patients with autonomic dysfunction and poor sleep tend to have a large number of spontaneous arousals, which appear to be directly related to autonomic dysfunction.

At the top of Figure 1 is a hypnogram showing sleep stages through the night. Although there is an underlying cycling through the various stages of sleep, superimposed on this is a large number of arousals, seen as vertical lines. The lower tracing shows the patient's heart rate, which should be a relatively flat line, but instead shows almost constant fluctuations, fluctuations which mirror the arousals in the tracing above.

Figure 1

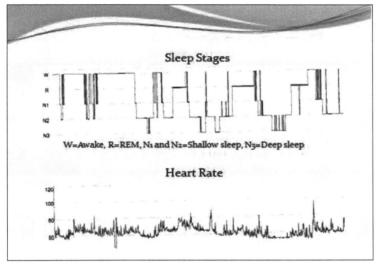

There are both pharmacologic and non-pharmacologic methods of reducing such "hyperarousal." Among the latter are relaxation techniques such as deep breathing, the effects of which can help patients fall asleep more easily, but which usually do not last more than a few hours. The mainstays of pharmacologic therapy are medications that either reduce sympathetic activity, i.e. alpha and beta blockers and clonidine and guanfacine; or medications that increase deep sleep, i.e. low-dose antidepressants such as trazodone, amitryptiline, and doxepin. Choosing the right drug or combination for each patient is largely a trial and error process, though patients who tend to get a "second wind" of energy in the evening tend to do better on a longer-acting beta blocker taken in the early evening, while others might need only a short acting beta blocker taken at bedtime. The alpha blocker prazosin tends to be particularly effective in patients who have frequent and/or vivid dreams.

Lastly, it is important not to overlook other factors which can adversely affect sleep quality, such as pain, depression, and anxiety, when developing a treatment regimen for dysautonomia patients with non-restorative sleep. Regimens that successfully reduce arousals and increase deep sleep almost without exception result in reductions in fatigue and improvements in well-being.

Dr. Pocinki is a general internist in private practice in Washington, D.C. His interest in Ehlers-Danlos and related autonomic and sleep problems over the past decade grew out of his experience studying chronic fatigue syndrome (CFS) since 1987. He has found that virtually all of his CFS patients (and fibromyalgia patients as well) have hypermobile joints, and autonomic and sleep problems similar to those of EDS patients. He has received a variety of awards and recognition for service to his 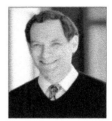 *profession, as well as for the quality of his practice, and speaks and writes regularly about these conditions. He is an Associate Clinical Professor at George Washington University School of Medicine and Health Sciences; and a Fellow of the American College of Physicians. He received his medical degree from Cornell University Medical College.*

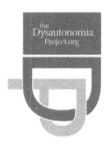

24

RESEARCH STUDY PARTICIPATION

by Bonnie Black, RN, ANP

There are a handful of academic medical centers in the United States that conduct research on the autonomic nervous system, including Vanderbilt in TN, Mayo Clinic in MN, the Harvard system in MA, New York University in NY, University of Texas in Dallas, TX, and the National Institutes of Health (NIH) in MD. Patients are recruited to participate in research. For a list of ongoing studies, visit *www.clinicaltrials.gov.*

Once you have been recruited for study participation, you and the research coordinator will select a mutually agreeable date for your screening visit. The screening could be separate from actual study participation, or it could be the initial part of the whole research experience.

The informed consent document is generally available in advance and is written in language that you should be able to understand. The reading level is purposefully chosen to be one that most readers can comprehend. You may need to review it a couple of times for details, but it should be very thorough about all aspects of the study. The format of the consent generally follows a template provided by the institution's Institutional Review Board, and it is reviewed and approved by a group of professionals in the conduct of human research. The consent form should be current and should include an approval date and an expiration date.

Every detail of the study should be outlined for you in the consent agreement. However, the coordinator is usually happy to outline in general terms how participation works and answer any questions. He or she would let you know a time frame for arrival to the unit and a general outline of your study days. Some studies are conducted during an inpatient stay, and others are outpatient studies and one comes and goes to the facility.

Ask the coordinator about appropriate clothing if she or he does not mention what to wear. The autonomic nervous system studies usually require the application of blood pressure cuffs, cardiac or other electrodes that are applied to the skin, and other recording devices. Casual, loose-fitting clothing is always appropriate. Bring a pair of slip-on shoes for walking down the hall in the hospital to protect your feet and allow for easy removal for the study. The investigator may specify shorts if they expose the upper leg during testing, as the appropriate garment allows easier access.

The study staff makes every attempt to recruit in advance patients or healthy controls that are appropriate for the study. They do this by reviewing outside records and, in some cases, make use of questionnaires. However, sometimes after the patient is selected it becomes clear the patient is not an ideal candidate for the study; then, a withdrawal takes place that could be the decision of the investigator or the subject. This is the best decision for all concerned, and is the best utilization of time and resources.

Whether you are staying at home or at a hotel, bring comfort items that help you get a good night's rest, such as a favorite blanket or pillow. Medical equipment, such as a C-pap machine, urinary catheters, and such, should be mentioned to the coordinator if you have any question about bringing your own.

Most autonomic studies do involve some discomfort due to study procedures. You should weigh your desire to participate with your actual clinical situation. Something as simple as lying quietly for several hours may be excruciating for a patient with chronic back pain. Blood samples that are a crucial part of a study may be almost impossible on a subject with a history of very poor intravenous access. A study that requires standing for periods of 10 minutes is not realistic for a patient who has been confined to bed for the past month. Patients can be both eager to help and desperate for help, and this may lead them to imagine they can comply with the rigors of a study when, realistically, they cannot. Discuss the described study procedures with the co-investigators and decide together if study participation is appropriate for you.

If you are fortunate to live in close proximity to a study center, travel there may not be time-consuming or difficult. Otherwise, it takes some planning. There may or not may not be funds to defray the cost of travel. If possible, plan to arrive early enough to be rested so you can start the screening process with a clear mind. Departure from the study center should be planned to allow for the appropriate rest needed to drive, fly, or otherwise travel home.

It is helpful to understand that the primary focus of a research study is to help the researchers learn more about a given condition. Their role is not to give you all the answers you have about your specific case. However, the researcher and the study results may help you and your doctor gain more knowledge about your condition, and this may help you devise an effective therapy program.

Bonnie K. Black, RN, ANP, BC graduated with a BSN from the University Of Nebraska Medical Center College of Nursing and earned her certification as an Adult Nurse Practitioner from an early program at the University of Vermont/VNA. She initially worked in cardiology and neurology for the Depart-ment of Veterans Affairs. She

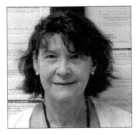

started the western VA Pacemaker Surveillance Program that provided trans-telephonic follow-up for veterans with implanted cardiac pacemakers. In 1994, she joined the faculty and staff of the Vanderbilt Autonomic Dysfunction Center, Vanderbilt University Medical Center as a research nurse. She recruits patients for studies in autonomic cardiovascular control from all over the United States and abroad.

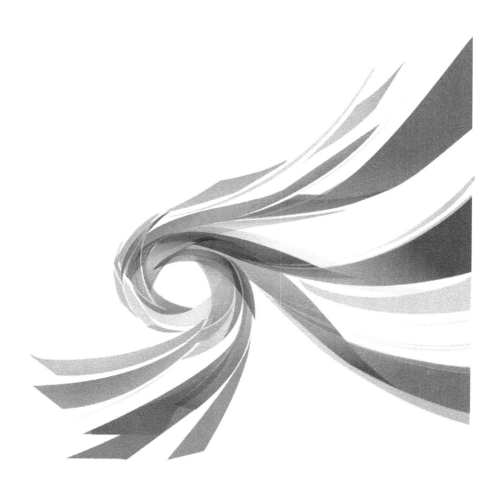

SECTION 4

MANAGING DYSAUTONOMIAS

A FEW THINGS EVERY PHYSICIAN, PATIENT, FRIEND, AND FAMILY MEMBER SHOULD KNOW

Knowledge is Power.

Francis Bacon
16th Century English Philospher

25

FLIP THE CLINIC*

FIND A GOOD PRIMARY DOCTOR AND BUILD THE RELATIONSHIP

Find a good doctor who can be your quarterback.

Ron Crown

Finding a good primary care doctor is an important achievement in ensuring you receive good health care. Like a football team has a quarterback who, along with the input of players and coaches, leads the play on the field, a good primary care doctor oversees the continuity of your care while working with you and other experts in the field.

A good primary care doctor:

- Is willing to learn with you about your condition (unless you are fortunate to have a primary care doctor who is also an autonomic specialist);

- Engages in a two-way conversation with you;

- Has ongoing follow-up appointments with you;

- Works with you to build a treatment plan, usually involving trial and error of different treatment options;

- Along with you, maintains copies of all your medical records;

- Works with you to ensure you gain access to appropriate care;

- May disagree with you at times, but explains why.

---

* Flip the Clinic is a Robert Wood Johnson Foundation program to improve the patient-clinician experience through collaboration.

25

FLIP THE CLINIC*

PHYSICIAN AND PATIENT COLLABORATION

Flip the Clinic is creating the possibility of a new system. It's creating a critical moment next to the 20 minute office visit that can be incredibly powerful for the delivery of health care and health.

Atul Gawande, MD, MPH

It is time to "flip the clinic." Patients with multi-system disorders of regulation, such as dysautonomias, should have more power and responsibility to manage their own health. Flip the clinic addresses this need. It is where patients and health care practitioners improve medical care, together.

The term "flip the clinic" refers to an initiative by the Robert Wood Johnson Foundation (RWJF) that encourages physicians and patients to work together to improve the patient-clinician experience. This book is a step in that direction because it provides a resource that both patients and clinicians can share. The Dysautonomia Project mission focuses on education to help flip the clinic, empowering and giving responsibility to patients with autonomic disorders. Learn more at *www.fliptheclinic.org.*

Flipping the clinic is an attempt to achieve two key goals. The first goal is to **empower patients, family, and caregivers** to be more informed and engaged in their own health and health care. The second goal is to **enable healthcare providers** to improve the ways they communicate with patients and support them better during and between office visits.

Most dysautonomia patients are treated poorly by community based health care practitioners today. The average POTS patient waits 6 years for a diagnosis, has seen over a dozen different doctors, and

Did you notice the phrase "with you" in each item on the list above? A good way to determine if you currently have a good primary care doctor is to ask the question, "Are they working 'with me' in taking care of my health?" If the answer is yes, you have a gem, and it is important to build that relationship.

Here are ways to build on that relationship:

- Be prepared for appointments. Bring information that updates the doctor on changes since your last visit and a list of questions you have.

- Ensure copies are sent to them from any specialists, hospitals you visit and all diagnostic tests. (Make sure you have your own copy too.)

- Recognize that the doctor has limited time and show appreciation if they spend extra time with you.

- Get to know members of the office staff and strive to build good relationship with them too.

- Keep in mind that your doctor is a scientist looking for facts to help you improve your health. Focus a majority of your appointment time on working together on ways to improve your health.

- If you need to go to the emergency room or get admitted to the hospital by a specialist, let them know. Keep them in the loop about any changes in your medical situation.

Not all doctors are a good fit with dysautonomia patients.

In the meantime, take comfort in knowing you are not alone. As these comments from dysautonomia patients or parents demonstrate, not all doctors are a good fit.

- *I can't count the number of times I've spent crying in the parking lot of a doctor's office after being treated badly. One time I cried for almost an hour after a doctor told me I should move out of this town and closer to a doctor who knows more about my condition.*

- *The pediatrician rolled his eyes at me when I tried to explain that I thought my daughter had dysautonomia.*

- *He said my condition was not life threatening, it was just a nuisance. Meanwhile, I can't drive or get out of bed most days.*

has been told by more than one physician that their condition is psychological in nature. To read comments made by patients about their experience with doctors, take a look at the end of the patient section of this chapter.

What many patients don't realize is that autonomic medicine is not taught well in medical education. As a physician you can help patients, but you will have more success if they are willing to work with you in sharing information, in determining if additional testing is needed, and in developing a treatment plan to manage their symptoms.

There is not one way or method to flip the clinic, but here are some ideas that may help you flip the clinic in your practice:

- Explain to the patient that in dysautonomias, especially complex cases, it is important to have a new mindset in the patient/physician relationship. It is essential that the patient not rely on you as having all the answers. Instead, you will work together to improve their health condition because no two cases of dysautonomia are exactly alike.

- Emphasize that the most important treatment for dysautonomia is education. Encourage patients to learn and understand their specific dysautonomia condition. Suggest they use internet-based learning, online patients support groups, and other resources.

- Ask them periodically about something new they have learned, or about lifestyle adjustments they have made that have been helpful.

- Coach patients and family members on using data, such as journaling symptoms, tracking medicine changes, etc. to make scientific decisions.

- When appropriate, suggest helpful technology resources, such as the mobile applications for tracking symptoms.

- Ask patients to report back on progress they make when trying a new treatment. If it is a drug with significant precautions, ask them to call in and report any adverse side effects within a few days of testing a new medication.

- *The doctor had a nurse talk with me and do an EKG. He then came in for 10 minutes and told me what he thought without asking me for more information. I got a bill for $450 for that appointment.*

- *My doctor said she couldn't find anything wrong with me and referred me to a counselor. She said it is all in my head.*

A good primary doctor is difficult to find. If you do not have a good primary care doctor, find one. This may require trying several doctors. Depending on where you live, you many need to travel an hour or two. Try to get recommendations from other dysautonomia patients and/or visit *www.TheDysautonomiaProject.org/Resources/5* for a growing physician list. Finding the right doctor for you is hard, but the effort is worth it.

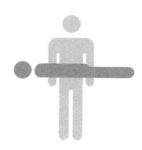

- Encourage patients to keep copies of all their medical records, and lab and diagnostic test results, and to organize them by date in a binder. When receiving lab or diagnostic results, ask them if they have a copy in their file.

- Use this book to have discussions with your patients and teach them about dysautonomia. Direct them to read the patient side of the book on their own.

From a scientific point of view, flipping the clinic will be especially valuable for patients with dysautonomia, a condition where the most important treatment is education.

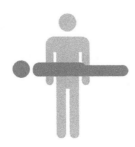

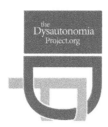

26

TOP ENEMIES OF DYSAUTONOMIA

Stress and Pain

by Charles R. Thompson, MD and Co-Author

One caveat before I begin this—for the sake of brevity I'll use "POTS" when referring to all forms of dysautonomia involving chronic orthostatic intolerance, whether POTS, neurally mediated syncope, idiopathic hypervolemia, etc. And, I'll be the first to admit, when I sat down to write this I was like, "well this will take two minutes and two lines." It seems obvious that stress and pain are the enemies. But bear with me, because when you talk about stress you think about a lot of different areas. I'm going to touch on some and how they affect us. And as you read, keep in mind, this is from somebody who is living with POTS.

Emotional Stress

Emotional stress affects you whether you are the CEO of a fortune 500 company, or bedbound and worrying about how you're going to make ends meet. Even people without POTS will have problems with stress, depression, alcoholism, drug abuse, etc. And if it's going to cause problems like that in a healthy person, imagine what it would do to your body. You are already fighting this fatigue, dyspnea, palpitations, nausea, and all the other symptoms of POTS, and now you throw emotional stress in the mix and the results are not good.

We have to face the fact we live in a world with tremendous emotional stress. And, it's going to affect your POTS worse than just about anything. So, there are some things you need to keep in mind. One, you're not going to get much sympathy from people who don't have POTS.

They have stressful lives, too. But, if you find yourself in a stressful situation, or know you're going to be in one, you'd better evaluate if a POTS episode is about to follow. Trouble is, everybody thinks of stress as all the bad things: financial problems, relationship problems, job problems, things of this nature. But you need to remember that stress is in everything. When you begin to consider stress, you have to think about things you don't really think about as being stressful. Good things--birthdays, vacations, holidays, family reunions. They're all great! But they're all stressful, and you need to be aware of it. What do you do about it? I've been dealing with it for 17 years, and when I figure it out, I'll let you know.

Pain

I considered putting this in several different categories because it encompasses so many different areas physical pain. Whether acute or chronic, it is going to really rev up the fight-or-flight mechanism. Again, going back to people who don't have POTS, look at how physical pain affects their lives. Now take POTS and then add pain on top of it--the results are not good. Both pain and POTS are making you release stress hor-

I tell all my patients that until we can at least get chronic and acute pain under control, we're probably not going to make much headway in treatment.

mones in your body, and your body can only handle so much. It can be any sort of pain, from chronic back pain to migraine headaches; it is going to affect your POTS, and it does have to be dealt with.

Atmospheric Stress

Have you figured out that we're better predictors of the weather than the people on TV? It's because of the effect the weather has on our bodies. I live in Pensacola, Florida, so I get a lot of strange looks when I tell people they need to avoid excessive heat. But as discussed in other chapters, the temperature plays a direct role in the pooling of the blood.

We already have the pooling of more blood in the legs and abdominal area then most non-POTS people. And the way your body gets rid of heat is to dilate blood vessels in the skin to give off heat to the atmosphere through perspiration. So then you have pooling of blood in the skin. And we have a lot of skin we can put blood into. People ask how I handle the heat. I tell them I can go from the air conditioning in my office, to the AC of my truck, to the AC at home. I have one neighbor who moved in several months ago who thinks I'm a vampire because he only sees me after the sun is down. Of course, I don't want patients trapped at home, but they have to pick their spots and try to stay out of the midday 100° heat and 100% humidity.

> *I have one neighbor who moved in several months ago who thinks I'm a vampire because he only sees me after the sun is down.*

I would also caution you that you can stay out of heat, but changes in barometric pressure are going to be a battle too. People think I'm joking, but I'm not. I can tell when a tropical front hits the Gulf, or if there is a front in Texas headed this way. And again, there's no way to avoid it. You have to give in to it or you'll end up on the floor.

Orthostatic and Other Physical Stress

Ever wonder why you can usually walk at a brisk clip but it's almost impossible to stand in one place very long? It all goes back to this pooling of the blood. Think about this. While you're still pooling blood in the abdominal area, you walk. Since the muscles in the legs act as a pump, they move the blood from your legs back up into the central circulation. This, in a way, takes the place of the blood pooling in the abdomen. But, if you stop and stand still, this muscle pumping stops and blood again pools in your legs. Since this blood comes away from the brain (not dangerously), you get very symptomatic. It sounds strange, but sitting is also an orthostatic position. When we sit, our brains are still higher than where our blood is pooling, so we'll again lose some blood flow to the brain and can get symptomatic. So standing or sitting in one place too long is not a good thing for us to do. One thing that will somewhat help us overcome this is using counter maneuvers. I'm not going to explain them here because they are covered in the chapter about non-pharmacological treatments.

Other things you may find strange might be explained by this pooling phenomenon. Bending over from the waist is a terrible position for us. Although we never pump our hearts dry, with the pooling of the blood we have less circulatory volume. When we bend over we increase the pressure in the chest and have less blood return to the heart, and when we stand back up the first few beats of our hearts don't supply as much blood flow to the brain as the brain wants, so we'll get dizzy. We could even pass out. Some of the worst motions we can do, and husband's usually want to kill me when I tell this part of it (remember this is about a 5 to 1 female to male ratio condition), but some of the worst motions are sweeping, mopping, vacuuming, and anything that involves working above the shoulder level. Why? Because, these motions restrict blood flow back to the chest. When people with POTS pass out, it's mostly in three places.

The Shower

The first is in the shower. When you shower you're probably doing 4 things you shouldn't do:

1. Standing still,
2. Lie if you want to, but you're under hot water (very few people enjoy taking cold showers),
3. You have your arms above your head working your hair and,
4. You're bending over to wash your feet and legs.

The Kitchen

The second place is in the kitchen. You're standing still and next to the heat of the stove, and it affects you. Or, you're loading or unloading the dishwasher, so you bend, you stand, and then you reach above your head to put the dishes away. And what happens when you do laundry? When you clean? I'm not trying to keep you from doing housework, but these hazards are why you can only do a little at a time and have to sit down.

Big Stores

One last example and you're through with me. It is almost impossible to do big store shopping trips. You park 2 miles away from the store and have to walk across the asphalt, which is radiating up heat. You're getting into an episode, but don't realize it, so you go into the store and get your buggy. By this time the fight-or-flight mechanisms are kicking in and, without you even thinking about it, you begin to focus inward, because everything else is sensory overload. The ceilings are high, the neon lights strobe. It's crowded. It's loud. Some child in the aisle over is getting his behind whooped (at least in backwoods Alabama where I grew up). You will walk 5 feet and stop, and walk 5 feet and stop. And then you bend down or reach above your head to get something and within five minutes your body is screaming. Leave

Pay attention to your body and your surroundings and "give in" when you have symptoms otherwise you're likely to end up on your nose.

the buggy. Leave everything and get out of there. If you don't, you probably won't like the consequences. You can read more in Chapter 7 about adrenaline and fight-or-flight stress response.

The takeaway message of this chapter is to pay attention to your body and your surroundings and "give in" when you have symptoms; otherwise, you're likely to end up on your nose in a place you don't want it to happen (not that you ever want it to happen).

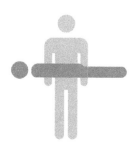

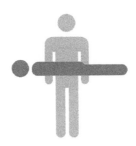

27

DEAR FAMILY MEMBERS & FRIENDS

PLEASE READ THIS

Dear family member or friend,

If the person you care about has been diagnosed with a form of dysautonomia (e.g. POTS, orthostatic hypotension, among others), they have a disorder of the autonomic (automatic) nervous system. Symptoms usually range from mild to disabling but, in some cases, can be life-threatening. Because most of the problems occur inside the body, dysautonomia is an "invisible illness." People with dysautonomia need your help.

- While they may look perfectly fine on the outside, even on their best days, the inside of their body is working overtime to maintain homeostasis, a healthy state of being.

- Some family members may think it's "all in their head," or they are "making this up." The truth is, dysautonomia is an internal medical condition that needs to be taken seriously.

- Plans may change. Your family member or friend may become very ill with symptoms at the last minute, just before a big night out or a special event, and they may not be able to attend. It's important that you are supportive and willing to be flexible when they don't feel well.

- Protect them from the enemies of dysautonomia, including stress and physical pain.

- Encourage healthy habits, such as appropriate exercise, diet, and sleep, in a way that does not increase their stress. (Exercise may help to improve function, but it is often difficult due to exercise intolerance and is not a cure for dysautonomia.)

- Recognize warning signs that indicate they might need to stop, slow down, or lie down. This may include exposure to heat, exercise, showers, and being in large crowds.

27

DEAR OFFICE STAFF

PLEASE READ THIS

Re: Patients with Dysautonomia

Dysautonomia, pronounced dis-auto-NO-mia, is a general term to describe a group of disorders of the autonomic (automatic) nervous system (e.g. POTS, orthostatic hypotension, among others). Symptoms usually range from mild to disabling but, in some cases, can be life-threatening. Because most of the problems occur inside the body, dysautonomia is an "invisible illness."

These patients may have a few special needs that may be helpful for you to be aware of, including:

- Most have difficulty standing, such as when at the counter waiting for check out. This is due to orthostatic intolerance or hypotension. Common symptoms include lightheadedness and syncope (fainting), so if you know a patient with dysautonomia will need to wait, you might offer them a chair so they can sit down.

- When helping with referrals, it is ideal if the specialist is familiar with dysautonomia. Most physicians don't learn about dysautonomia in medical school and some treatments are counterintuitive. For example, a diet high in fiber is often mistakenly recommended, but this can exacerbate blood pooling and actually worsen symptoms because it shunts too much blood away from vital organs. If your office sees many dysautonomia patients, you might start an office referral list of other physicians in your area who are familiar with dysautonomia.

- If a patient arrives or becomes symptomatic and the physician is not immediately available, have the patient lie down, drink water and, if possible, eat something salty (unless they tend to

- They may not be able to do all the things they used to do, including shopping, household chores, and attending big parties.

You can help by learning more about dysautonomia, and by protecting them from people who do not understand. It helps to:

- Ask them how they are feeling and genuinely listen.
- Remind them that you are there to support them and that you're not going anywhere.
- Sit in on appointments with doctors, if appropriate.
- Avoid saying things such as:

  You look so good you must be feeling better.

  If you would only _____ (lose weight, exercise, or any other fill in the blank) you would get better.

  If you just have a positive attitude and put your mind to it you can push through the symptoms.

Statements like these might not only hurt feelings, but they might also push the person you care about into overdoing it, which can be harmful to their health.

Patients with dysautonomia are at a triple disadvantage.

1. Most people have never heard of it.
2. Most doctors were not well trained about dysautonomia in medical school.
3. It's an invisible illness, so it's easy for other people to say things that are insensitive even though they might mean well.

Your family member or friend is facing a difficult medical battle. There is no cure for dysautonomia. Treatments are aimed at managing symptoms and improving function, where possible. It often takes time to find the right doctors and combination of treatments to improve health. The people who have this condition may struggle with feelings of anxiety or depression, especially when they experience episodes involving difficult symptoms. They need your support in facing the days ahead.

On behalf of The Dysautonomia Project,

Kelly

Kelly Freeman, MSM
Founding Director, The Dysautonomia Project
www.TheDysautonomiaProject.org

be hypertensive) until the doctor is available.

Your extra consideration for dysautonomia patients is appreciated. Learn more about dysautonomia at *www.TheDysautonomiaProject.org*

Sincerely,

Kelly

Kelly Freeman, MSM
Founding Director, The Dysautonomia Project
www.TheDysautonomiaProject.org

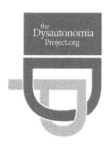

28

POTS & DEPRESSION

AN INVISIBLE ILLNESS AFFECTS THE BODY AND THE MIND

by Kelly Freeman, MSM and Co-author

Postural orthostatic tachycardia syndrome (POTS) is a common but rarely known health condition affecting an estimated 1 in 100 teenagers and, in the United States, as many as 3 million adult and teen patients combined.[1] One of the most common forms of dysautonomia, POTS, is a dysfunction of the autonomic (or automatic) nervous system that involves abnormal symptoms in many parts of the body, including abnormal blood flow to the heart, lungs, and brain. It often involves problems with digestion, temperature regulation, and many other involuntary functions of the body. Because the condition involves the autonomic nervous system, which regulates mostly internal functions, it is commonly known as an "invisible illness."

This chronic condition can be mild to disabling in patients. Just as a short in a light bulb can cause the light to go on sometimes and flicker off at other times, the electrical impulses of the nervous system in POTS patients work, or fail to work, in a similar way. Most POTS patients experience periods of time when the severity of their symptoms, and the levels of their pain, vary. In some patients, symptoms are mild for months at a time and then become severe for months. Other patients have symptoms that vary as frequently as hour to hour. Approximately 25% of POTS patients experience symptoms so severe that they are unable to attend school, work, and/or drive, and some are bedridden.

Because the person with POTS often cannot do the things healthy people can do, and must also deal with the vast lack of understanding of POTS in both the general population and the medical field, signs of depression in POTS patients are common. While further study is needed to clearly understand the relationship between psychological conditions such as depression and its relationship to POTS, three research teams, from Vanderbilt University, The National Institutes of Health, and Baker IDI Heart & Diabetes Institute in Melbourne, VIC, Australia, have helped us begin to better understand this relationship. Four trends seem to be emerging from recent medical literature:

1. POTS is a mind-body disorder. It is a condition with both physiological and psychological symptoms that are caused, in part, by the abnormal release of chemical mediators, known as neurotransmitters, in the brain and other parts of the body.

2. Most patients with POTS have pronounced cognitive difficulties, such as inattention, which appear to be more pronounced in severity than symptoms of anxiety and/or depression.

3. Symptoms of POTS, including cognitive function, anxiety, and depression, are worsened by stress, including physical stress, such as orthostatic (upright) stress, and emotional stress.

4. Neurotransmitters such as norepinephrine, dopamine, adrenaline, serotonin and acetylcholine, which help the nervous system work, are often released abnormally in patients with POTS and can affect the mental state of the POTS patient.

It is important to use caution, especially initially, when taking antidepressant medications such as SSRIs [2] or SNRIs [3], or other medications such as epinephrine, which is often used in local anesthetics. These medications can further change the balance of the chemical neurotransmitters that are used by the nervous system.

In a Vanderbilt Autonomic Dysfunction Center Study conducted in 2008, that compared POTS patients with both ADHD patients and a normal control group, researchers revealed:

Patients with POTS did not have an increased prevalence of major depression or anxiety disorders, including panic disorder, compared with the general population. Patients with POTS had mild depression. They scored as moderately anxious on the Beck Anxiety Inventory, but did not exhibit a high level of anxiety sensitivity. Patients with POTS scored significantly higher on inattention and ADHD subscales than control subjects. These symptoms were not present during childhood. Patients with POTS do not have an increased lifetime prevalence of psychiatric disorders. Although they may seem anxious, they do not have excess cognitive anxiety. They do experience significant inattention, which may be an important source of disability."[4]

> Patients with POTS do not have an increased lifetime prevalence of psychiatric disorders.

In Australia, researchers studied cognition, anxiety, and depression during the tilt table test and found acute changes in mental ability when the patients were in an upright position:

Acute changes in cognitive performance in response to head up tilt were evident in the POTS patients. It was concluded that participants with POTS have an increased prevalence of depression and higher levels of anxiety. These underlying symptoms impact on cognition in patients with POTS, particularly in the cognitive domains of attention and short-term memory.[5]

David S. Goldstein, MD, PhD, Senior investigator at the National Institute of Neurological Disorders and Stroke, explains how dysautonomias involve both the physical and mental health of the patient:

Disorders involving the adrenaline family are, possibly more than any other ailments, mind-body disorders. In many ways the autonomic nervous system operates exactly at the border of the mind and body. This is a difficult subject for both doctors and patients. The problem is the old notion that the body and mind are separate and distinct in a person and so disease must be either physical or mental. If the disorder were physical it would be "real," something imposed on the individual, whereas if it were mental, and "in your head," it would not be real, but something created in and by the individual... (these notions) are outdated.[6]

It is appropriate to note that some patients with POTS have coexisting conditions that add complexity to their cases. The research reference listed above isolated patients with a confirmed diagnosis of POTS without other coexisting medical conditions.

In managing their condition, patients with POTS experience a three-pronged battle: the physical, the emotional, and the spiritual. Clearly there are many physical difficulties that must be managed, such as dealing with abnormal circulation and the abnormal response to the stress of an upright posture. As mentioned in the research above, there are also many emotional/mental difficulties to overcome. Additionally, there is the spiritual battle, which, if ignored can, in part, cause the POTS patient to "lose hope."

According to Harvard Medical School trained author and practicing psychiatrist, Doug Welpton, MD, there is an important distinction to be made between depression and despair. Despair is depression at its worst. When a person's depression becomes despair, the person has lost hope. [7] If people are depressed, they may seem tired, lack initiative, and have low energy. But, if people who are exhibiting signs of depression "give up" or "lose hope," they may have reached a stage where they may

> Dysautonomia is a physical, emotional, and spiritual battle.

become a danger to themselves and/or to others. It is important to note that many POTS patients consider the thought of dying as an alternative to the reality of suffering. But, most do not report thoughts about planning a suicide.

If you are concerned about depression in yourself or someone you know who has POTS, seek the help of a licensed medical professional who is knowledgeable about dysautonomia.

The POTS patient who has a high level of stress, a lack of support from family and friends in dealing with their condition, and who is not connected with medical professionals who can guide them in managing their invisible illness is at the highest risk for losing hope.

The best way to keep depression from turning into despair is to fight the three-pronged battle. Fight physically by gaining knowledge of POTS and finding medical professionals who are willing to have a two-way discussion, who will work together with you to create and adapt treatment plans as needed. Fight emotionally to feel loved and supported by family members and friends who understand the unique needs of the POTS patient. Help them understand your need to sometimes talk openly about your symptoms and about how much it helps you when they are flexible, especially when your symptoms become more severe. And, finally, fight spiritually to have faith in a greater power that gives both strength and hope.

[1] Dysautonomia International Webpage; What is Dysautonomia? March 11, 2015

[2] Mar, Philip L. et. al. "Acute Hemodynamic Effects of a Selective Serotonin Reuptake Inhibitor in Postural Orthostatic Tachycardia Syndrome: A Randomized Crossover Trial." *Journal of Psychopharmacology* (Oxford, England) November 13, 2013.

[3] Green, Elizabeth A. et. al. "Effects of Norepinephrine Reuptake Inhibition on Postural Orthostatic Tachycardia Syndrome." *Journal of The American Heart Association*; October 2, 2013.

[4] Raj, V. et. al., "Psychiatric profile and Attention Deficits in Postural Tachycardia Syndrome." *Journal of Neurology, Neurosurgery & Psychiatry*; October 31, 2008.

[5] Anderson, Jake W. et. al., "Cognitive Function, Health-Related Quality of Life, and Symptoms of Depression and Anxiety Sensitivity are Impaired in Patients with the Postural Orthostatic Tachycardia Syndrome (POTS). *Frontiers in Physiology*. June 25, 2014.

[6] Goldstein, David S. *Adrenaline and the Inner World: An Introduction to Scientific Integrative Medicine*. Johns Hopkins University Press, Baltimore, MD; 2006

[7] Welpton, Doug. Phone Interview. March 12, 2015.

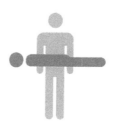

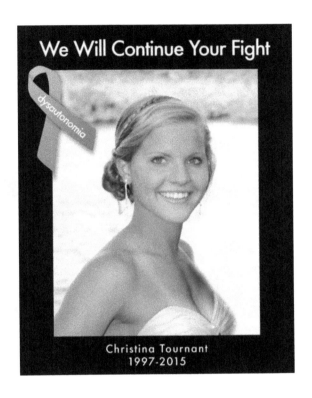

We Will Continue Your Fight

dysautonomia

Christina Tournant
1997-2015

This chapter was written in memory of Christina Tournant (June 24, 1997—March 5, 2015), who impacted the lives of so many people. We will continue your fight.

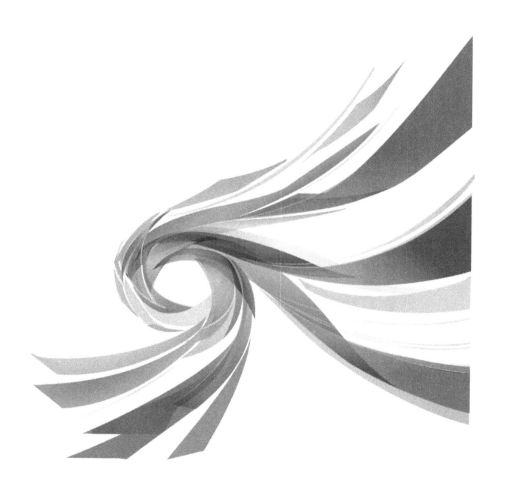

SECTION 5

TREATMENT OPTIONS

MANAGING DYSAUTONOMIA

Organs are made for action, not existence;
they are made to work, not to be; and
when they work well, they can be well.

Henry Hyde Salter, English physician,
author, *On Asthema, 1864*

29

THE #1 TREATMENT IS EDUCATION

The Responsible and Well-Educated Patient

Dysautonomia often requires the patient to become the scientist.
Italo Biaggioni, MD
Autonomic Research Center
Vanderbilt University

Learning about dysautonomia as a patient often begins just after diagnosis with how to pronounce "dysautonomia" (dis-auto-NO-mia). And, in most cases, it becomes an ongoing process of putting together bits and pieces of information like a gigantic jigsaw puzzle.

Dysautonomia is unlike the vast majority of other patient conditions, such as diabetes, cardiovascular disease, or appendicitis where:

- the doctor is the expert,
- treatment plans are fairly similar, and
- the patient's main job is to show up for appointments and follow the doctor's orders.

In dysautonomia, often the local doctor is not an expert in disorders of the autonomic nervous system. There is not a universal treatment plan that meets the needs of all patients, and trial and error of different drugs and non-pharmacological treatments is often necessary to achieve meaningful improvement in symptoms. Therefore, it is important that patients become well educated about their condition and work collaboratively with their doctor(s) to develop a meaningful treatment plan.

The goal for most dysautonomia patients is not necessarily to return to full health, but to learn how to gradually have more good days than

29

THE #1 TREATMENT
IS EDUCATION

PHYSICIAN AS A FACILITATOR OF
THE SCIENTIFIC PROCESS

No single therapy is uniformly successful...
Dysautonomia Information Network
2015

Successful management of dysautonomia involves more than obtaining a correct diagnosis and then instituting curative treatment. Even in the most sophisticated and knowledgeable centers, the diagnosis remains uncertain, especially for functional disorders. Even an agreed upon diagnosis, such as postural orthostatic tachycardia syndrome, does not necessarily carry with it agreed upon ideas about the mechanism of the condition, the most appropriate treatment, or the long-term outcome.

Dwelling on finding "cures" for dysautonomias is unrealistic. Instead, focus on understanding the etiology of the specific case so you can best select therapies to consider as a part of the treatment plan.

There are many treatments for dysautonomias, including non-drug and drug treatments, and there are many coping tactics. This section focuses on these aspects of autonomic medicine.

While most dysautonomias require clinical management, it is important to note that some forms of dysautonomia are either episodic or secondary. In cases where the dysautonomia is episodic, such as reflex syncope, there is little need for ongoing clinical management. Where the dysautonomia is secondary to another condition, such as diabetes as is seen in diabetic autonomic neuropathy (DAN), managing the pri-

bad days by improving their ability to live life to its fullest while managing symptoms. In order to do this it is helpful to:

1) Read about dysautonomia from books, articles, and websites, including *www.TheDysautonomiaProject.org*.

2) Keep a journal of your medications and symptoms, making note of what seems to help, and what seems to worsen symptoms or cause side effects. (There are several mobile apps to help with managing your health and keeping track of symptoms. One for the iPhone we've tried and like is called "Symple.")

3) Participate in online discussions with other patients who have similar symptoms. Avoid groups that have participants who spend a lot of time complaining about their symptoms. Look for groups where you can ask questions and learn from others. A few we recommend are: *www.DINET.org/patient forum*; Dysautonomia Advocacy Foundation Facebook group; and The Dysautonomia Project (TDP) Facebook page and/or local TDP Facebook group.

4) Go back to school or focus school studies on the biological sciences so that you can better understand medical terms and the various systems within the human body.

5) When working with a physician to develop a treatment plan:

   • Make only one change at a time so that you can determine if the treatment change is truly helpful. (That might be a new drug, a new dosage, a new exercise plan, a dietary change, etc.)

   • Keep a list of current medications and dosages, including a list of all medications tried previously and discontinued with an explanation of why each was discontinued.

   • Periodically consider taking a "drug holiday" (a week or two off) from each of your regular medications to ensure each continues to be effective. Of course, it is important to consult your physician before making any changes or taking a break from your medications.

   • Think of yourself as a scientist on a mission to find the best set of pharmacological and/or non-pharmacological treatments. Use the scientific method and data to make decisions with your physician(s).

mary condition should be the main focus while use of treatments to aid autonomic neuropathy symptoms are supplemental.

For those dysautonomias where greater clinical management is needed, it is helpful to establish a rhythm of follow-up appointments with the patient where the trial and error aspects of various treatments are considered, tested, and documented. This "Flip the Clinic" approach positions the physician as the facilitator of the scientific process, and it engages the patient in regularly reporting on symptoms after the trial of new treatments. When adopted effectively, this approach creates:

- A meaningful dialogue about the effectiveness or ineffectiveness of various treatments; and

- Gives both patient and provider hope that with time and persistence improvement in symptoms will occur.

Most patients will need some coaching on how to test various treatments, document symptoms, and collaborate scientifically in developing an effective treatment plan. Here is a list of helpful tips in becoming a strong facilitator of the scientific process with your patients.

List of Tips in Facilitating the Scientific Process with Patients
Remind patients we have a long list of treatment options available. With time and persistence, most patients have improvement in symptoms.
Teach the basics of the scientific method. In order to determine if a drug or other treatment is effective, we can only change one variable at time.
Say the same thing each time you see the patient, "I'm counting on you to keep good records and report back to me."
I often say, "This is a Marathon, not a Sprint."
Before you enter the exam room have the nurse check which treatments have been tested since the patient's last appointment.

* This list has been created by The Dysautonomia Project physicians and patient advisors. It may grow or change based on feedback. Check our website for the most updated "List of Tips" at www.TheDysautonomiaProject.org/Resources/6.

30

NON-PHARMACOLOGICAL TREATMENTS

The rhythmic contractions of the leg muscles,
called the "muscle pump," act as a second heart.
Frank Rosato
Walking & Jogging for Health & Wellness

In considering the following treatments it is important to understand that the aim of the following treatments is to improve function and reduce symptoms. If someone says, "If only you would lose weight", or "If only you would exercise more" and thinks you will be cured, he/she might mean well, but they are wrong. A healthy diet and exercise program is beneficial for everyone, including patients with dysautonomia, but alone it is not a cure.

Salt and Water

Salt, also known as sodium, is an electrolyte. Its main job is to help the body keep a proper balance of fluid and electrolytes. There is a saying in the medical world: water always follows salt. This is because the body wants to keep a specific ratio of salt to water. It strives for equilibrium, homeostasis.

When you are dehydrated you do not have enough water in your body. Urine becomes darker since there is less water diluting it. The body wants to keep the perfect ratio of sodium to water. In a dehydrated state, a specific hormone signals the body to retain water and excrete more sodium. Drinking more water will help to restore the right balance of water to sodium content in your body. If you have too much water, your urine will be light. Light or clear urine is an indicator that your body is getting rid of excess water to restore the correct ratio.

30

NON-PHARMACOLOGICAL TREATMENTS

I was at an autonomic conference at Mayo with nine leading autonomic doctors in a round table discussion. The question was asked, "If you had a patient on a deserted island what one thing would you give them?" They all said, "water." One said, "Salt water." One said, "Live in the water."

Randy Thompson, MD

Some of the most important treatments for patients with dysautonomia don't involve the use of medications. Treatment should be aimed at:

- Controlling the pooling of blood in the lower parts of the body
- Staying hydrated
- Keeping heart rate and blood pressure under control
- Avoiding stress and pain

Salt and Water

Sodium plays a significant role in combating orthostatic intolerance. An increase of sodium in the diet has been shown to aid in better sympathetic nervous system regulation of vasoconstriction and cerebral autoregulation.[1] Sodium along with water in the proper ratio increases the overall fluid volume in the body, but does not significantly impact resting blood pressure.

Water also creates a pressor response in dysautonomia patients. This response peaks 20 minutes after water is ingested and increases peripheral vascular resistance, which attenuates fall in stroke volume. In postural orthostatic tachycardia syndrome, water has been shown to decrease orthostatic tachycardia. In patients with pure autonomic failure, water intake helps lessen orthostatic hypotension and post meal drops in blood pressure.[2]

Conversely, when more sodium is ingested, it triggers the thirst mechanism and the consumption of water. The water joins the extra salt and helps restore the balance of water and salt.

Increasing fluid volume increases pressure in the vascular system, including the pressure in veins and arteries. When your body is dehydrated, fluid increase can help return low blood pressure back to normal. At that range your heart does not have to work as hard. This can be illustrated using a hose. Using a one-inch hose instead of a three-inch hose can increase the pressure. The smaller diameter causes the water to shoot out with greater force. Just as the narrower hose creates more pressure, certain medications can also cause narrowing of the veins and arteries. This is called vasoconstriction. Salt is needed to help the body hold on to water. Greater sodium in the diet along with increased water intake, maintains equilibrium while increasing blood pressure. Just increasing one of these things puts the body out of balance and mechanisms must counteract this, as discussed above. Dysautonomia patients should increase salt in their diet, unless they experience high blood pressure. The general rule with most dysautonomia patients is to salt food as much as tolerable.[1]

Up to 10 grams (about two teaspoons) of salt a day is recommended for dysautonomia patients who do not have high blood pressure. A helpful technique is to measure this amount in a small bowl and use as much as you can throughout the day, gradually increasing your consumption until you are consistently getting the targeted amount. Alternatively, salt tablets can be used to supplement.

The daily-recommended water intake is two to four liters, spread out over a day. At least half of the daily fluid intake should be rich in electrolytes, such as Gatorade™, NUUN™ tablets, or Smart Water™. This can also be achieved economically by drinking water and ingesting salt separately.

Energy drinks and alcohol should be used with caution or avoided due to their dehydrating nature and their effect on the heart and nervous system. Carbonated beverages should be ingested sparingly, or not at all, as the body must work to expel the extra carbon dioxide ingested. This is why many professional athletes limit or avoid them.

An increase in both salt and water intake is recommended for patients with orthostatic intolerance or orthostatic hypotension. It is not recommended for patients who experience hypertension or those with certain comorbidities. It is important to try to keep the correct electrolyte balance. It is recommended that patients drink two to four liters spread out over 24 hours. Patients with gastroparesis often have a difficult time ingesting the daily amount of needed fluid. Sodium chloride IV therapy may be a needed supplementation. It is important to avoid IV infusions that are too frequent. The amount at which IV fluids become too much may vary from patient to patient. Patients should ingest as much salt as they can handle, with a target amount of ten grams a day. Fludrocortisone can be used to help the kidneys retain this extra sodium and thereby raise fluid volume more effectively.

Exercise

Exercise should be stressed and considered as one of the most important treatments for dysautonomia. Patients with dysautonomia often have a significant degree of deconditioning that occurs, which worsens symptoms. Exercise routines must be customized for each patient. It is important to find an exercise option the patient can enjoy, tolerate, and keep up with. This needs to be followed up with and stressed at every appointment. Low recumbent exercise has been shown to be the most tolerated. Aerobic exercise can improve cardiac output and thereby decrease stroke volume, leading to a decrease in heart rate. Exercise also strengthens the muscles, improves vascular tone, and helps with circulation.

> *Exercise is one of the most important activities for dysautonomia patients and should be part of every treatment plan.*

Atrophy of the muscles and joints is another enemy of dysautonomia due to inactivity or comorbidities. Keeping patients active is key. Wheelchairs should only be used on a regular basis as a last resort, as it will worsen both deconditioning and atrophy. Patients with Ehlers-Danlos syndrome should not be instructed to stretch. Special exercise considerations should be made for this comorbid condition. Post-exertional malaise and mountain sickness may occur when dysautonomia patients

Caffeine can be helpful for its energy boosting and blood vessel tightening effects. Some patients find a high caffeine diet essential to their daily routine while others cannot tolerate increased caffeine. Caffeine is a diuretic; so for every cup of caffeine, consider ingesting one cup of water to balance the loss of fluids from the body.

Exercise

Exercise is perhaps one of the most important treatments of dysautonomia. Being out of shape significantly worsens your symptoms. Exercise lowers your heart rate, strengthens your heart, and improves the tone of your vascular system. In patients with chronic pain, exercise helps by releasing endorphins, chemicals your body creates naturally which improves overall pain. It is important to stay active, as inactivity not only worsens your symptoms but causes your muscles and joints to break down. An individualized exercise plan is key. Find exercise that is tolerable, enjoyable, and that you can do regularly. Joining friends or using an exercise trainer for accountability and enjoyment is recommended. Recumbent aerobic exercises, including swimming, rowing, and recumbent bike riding, are best tolerated in patients with dysautonomia. It is important that you take exercise as seriously as medication in the treatment of your condition.

Compression Garments

Compression hose and abdominal binders can help keep your blood from pooling. The pooling of blood in the abdomen or legs often causes dizziness or fainting in patients with dysautonomia. When you purchase compression hose, find those that are waist high and have a label that lists a compression of 30-40mmHg, which is how tight the compression is. Abdominal binders should be ones that are stepped into and not those that tie around the waste. Spanx™ is a good option. You should especially wear compression hose while you are exercising. Wearing compression sleeves for on your arms may also be useful. And you might benefit from abdominal binders and compression hose while traveling. Compression garments should be removed while at rest.

Diet and Supplements

Dysautonomia patients should eat small frequent meals. Large meals worsen dizziness because they shunt up to 5 times more blood into the abdominal area. Most patients do well to "graze" throughout the exercise. Patients who also have chronic fatigue syndrome may find exercise especially difficult. For patients with postural orthostatic tachycardia syndrome, target heart rate and maximum heart rate should be explained and a goal agreed upon and reviewed periodically.

Compression Garments

Compression garments help to lessen or prevent the pooling of blood, combating orthostatic hypotension and orthostatic intolerance. Abdominal binders, such as Spanx™, help with pooling in the splanchic bed. Abdominal binders should not be the kind that wrap around but the kind that require stepping into. Compression hose are helpful for blood pooling of the legs, especially during exercise. Compression sleeves for the arms may also be helpful for exercise. It is recommended that compression hose be 30-40mmHg and waist high. The combination of compression hose and an abdominal binder has been shown to be helpful for travel. They should be removed when at rest.

Diet and Supplements

Large meals trigger the shunting of blood to the GI system. This leads to an increase in postprandial orthostatic hypotension and orthostatic intolerance. Small frequent meals are recommended. For patients with severe dizziness and syncope after meals, low fiber diets may be something else to consider, as large amounts of fiber also divert blood flow to the gut. Reducing sugar and carbohydrates in the diet has been shown to be beneficial, as large amounts of these can worsen symptoms. Artificial foods, including those with dyes and preservatives, can also make patients feel worse. Patients with mast cell activation especially have difficulty with these additives. Healthy diets should be pursued, with avoidance of high fat content and processed foods. Patients should seek whole and organic foods. Patients with gastroparesis and the poor GI motility often experience nausea and/or find adherence to a proper diet difficult. Protein shakes and drinks without a milk base, such as Ensure Clear, are usually tolerable. Options such as TPN and PN should be used a last resort. Pre-albumin levels should be monitored in dysautonomia patients as a helpful assessment of diet.

It is common for dysautonomia patients to be deficient in vitamins such as D, B6, and B12. Vitamin levels should be drawn periodically. In

day and save their larger meal for before bed. If you eat a big starchy meal, look for the couch. Some patients find it helpful to start the day with at least a little protein, such as a boiled egg or yogurt.

Large meals and high fiber foods redirect more blood to the gut, leaving less blood for other organs, such as the brain. This causes worsened symptoms after eating, sometimes resulting in postprandial (after eating) orthostatic hypotension.

Many patients find it helpful to reduce:

- Sugar
- High carbohydrates
- High fiber (except in the evening)
- Fast food / or highly processed foods
- Artificial foods, added chemicals and dyes

Consider a healthy, colorful diet of whole foods with cooked rather than raw vegetables, as cooked vegetables are easier for the body to digest. If you have a sluggish or paralyzed gastrointestinal system, consider low sugar, green juices, or non-milk based protein drinks such as Ensure Clear, as milk based drinks often exacerbate GI symptoms.

Counter Maneuvers

Your legs are like your second heart. They help to pump blood back into circulation. Many people who are unaware they have dysautonomia have used this "second heart" without realizing it during the counter maneuver techniques they employ to move around.

Many symptoms may occur when there is blood pooled in the legs and/or abdominal area. Crossing your legs while seated and squeezing the thigh muscles when standing can help combat this. Also try elevating your feet while seated. If you have to stand in line, hold onto something and do calf raises or tighten your buttocks to keep blood from pooling. Sleeping with the head of the head of the bed raised has been reported to help with morning dizziness. Using a seat in the shower is recommended, as showers exacerbate many dysautonomia symptoms. Seat canes are portable and useful for those who cannot handle prolonged standing.

---

[1] Hachul, D. (2014). "Does non-pharmacological treatment affect outcomes in dysautonomic syndromes?" *Cardiol J Cardiology Journal*, 21(6), 611-615.

patients with gastroparesis this can be an especially common finding. While giving mega-doses of vitamins is against RDA, it has been shown that oral ingestion of high doses of these vitamins can bypass the malabsorptive gut by osmosis into the blood stream.[3]

Counter maneuvers are maneuvers such as bending at the waist, crossing the legs while seated, and contracting the thighs. These increase peripheral resistance and act to reduce venous capacity.[4] Elevating the feet helps to prevent venous pooling while seated. Sleeping with the head of the bed raised has been shown to help morning orthostatic hypotension and intolerance. Using a shower seat can be suggested, as there is often significant venous pooling due to the combination of heat and orthostatic posture. Seat canes may be handy, especially for those who experience orthostatic intolerance.

[1,2,3] Hachul, D. (2014). Does non-pharmacological treatment affect outcomes in dysautonomic syndromes? Cardiol J Cardiology Journal, 21(6), 611-615.

[4] Low, P. A., & Singer, W. (2008). Update on Management of Neurogenic Orthostatic Hypotension. Lancet Neurology, 7(5), 451–458. doi: 10.1016/S1474-4422(08)70088-7

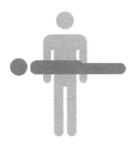

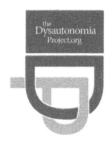

31

TOP 10 NON-PHARMACOLOGICAL TREATMENTS*

Several non-pharmacological treatments are used to help patients with dysautonomia. Although these treatments do not involve medicine, patients should discuss the use of such therapies with their physician as a part of the treatment plan.

Treatment	Helps with	Notes
Education	Patient being the advocate for his or her own care over time results in improvements in overall health. Selecting the right doctor to work with in managing your case is essential.	Don't just show up for appointments and expect your doctor to have all the answers. Engage in a two-way discussion.
Exercise	Confidence, vascular tone, large muscle strength, and release of pain fighting endorphins.	Must adjust for specific patient needs. Ideal to work with physical therapist to start.
Fluids	Prevents dehydration, and can create a helpful pressor effect.	Target 2-4 liters per day.
Salt	An essential electrolyte, which helps with nervous system function and effects blood pressure.	Up to 10 grams daily in moderate to low hypotensive patients.
Counter maneuvers	Act as a back-up heart, pumping blood that has pooled back into circulation.	A common sign of patients with dysautonomia.

Diet	Eat several small meals throughout the day to maintain glucose levels and postprandial hypotension.	Avoid: Highly processed foods with chemical additives.
Compression Garments	Prevent pooling of blood in lower parts of the body. Especially helpful in hypotensive patients.	Mid-thigh shaper Spanx™ known to increase systolic blood pressure by 10-15 mmHg in some patients.
Good Sleep Hygiene	Restorative sleep. Healing of the body and minimizes stress. Avoid stimulating activities 30 minutes prior to sleep.	Discuss any sleep issues with your physician.
Dietary Supplements including: Vitamins B-12 and Vitamin D	Vitamin supplementation can be especially important when essential vitamin levels are deficient. Vitamins B-12 and Vitamin D are sometimes low in patients with dysautonomia.	Recommend discussing any dietary supplements with your physician.
Cranio-Sacral /Manual Therapy	Increasing relaxation and reducing stress with a light touch therapy in regions of the spinal cord associated with parasympathetic nerves.	Some evidence that heart rate variability may improve. More research is needed.

* This top 10 list may change based on feedback of The Dysautonomia Project members and advisors. Check our website for the most updated top 10 list at: www.TheDysautonomiaProject.org/Resources/7.

32

PHARMACOLOGICAL TREATMENTS

Here is an overview of common drugs used in treating various forms of dysautonomia. A top 20 list can be found at the end of this chapter and on The Dysautonomia Project website.

Fludrocortisone (Florinef®)

Fludrocortisone is a steroid that helps the body retain salt. Salt is what helps the body retain water. This increase in "water weight" helps patients have increased blood volume. An increased blood volume helps keep a dysautonomia patient from experiencing drops in blood pressure when standing.

Fludrocortisone can cause low potassium levels. Your potassium level will need to be evaluated periodically, by a blood draw. This medication can also cause high blood pressure, especially when you are lying down. When used over the course of several months, this may help improve the pooling of blood in the abdominal area. Common side effects of fludrocortisone include difficulty sleeping, lightheadedness, headache, appetite changes, nausea, increased sweating, and nervousness.

It is important to increase dietary salt intake when taking fludrocortisone, as this medicine requires sodium to work effectively.

Midodrine (Proamatine®)

Midodrine is used to prevent low blood pressure. This drug also tightens blood vessels. This can be explained with the analogy of a garden hose. When you shrink the opening of the spout by placing your thumb over part of the opening, the water sprays out with much more force. This is what happens with tightened, or constricted, blood vessels. Blood can be circulated more easily because of the narrowing, just like with the hose.

32

PHARMACOLOGICAL TREATMENTS

Drugs that affect the production, release, or inactivation of catecholamines, or that work by stimulating or blocking receptors for catecholamines, are mainstays in the pharmacological treatment of various forms of dysautonomia. This chapter focuses on the most commonly used dysautonomia drugs. The top 20 drug list follows.

Fludrocortisone (Florinef®)

Fludrocortisone is the most commonly prescribed medication for dysautonomias involving orthostatic intolerance and orthostatic hypotension. It is a salt-retaining steroid or mineralocorticoid. It acts to retain sodium in exchange for potassium. Due to the increase in sodium, the patient gains "water weight" and blood pressure increases. This drug is thought to increase overall blood volume.

The downside of fludrocortisone is that it wastes potassium in exchange for sodium. Potassium levels must be carefully monitored, as hypokalemia can result. This drug can also cause exaggerated supine hypertension.[1] Fludrocortisone is not recommended for patients prone to hypertensive episodes. Fludrocortisone accelerates the progression of renal damage in Familial Dysautonomia.[2] Long-term use of fludrocortisone helps to up-regulate the norepinephrine receptors in the splanchnic bed so they bind the NE more effectively, improving vasoconstriction in the abdominal region.[3] Fludrocortisone is thought to be safer in low doses as higher does can suppress adrenal activity.[4] Fludrocortisone is most effective in combination with a high sodium diet.

Midodrine (Proamatine®)

Midodrine is the second most commonly prescribed drug for dysautonomia. It is an anti-hypotensive drug that works as a vasoconstrictor. This works well for blood pooling as a result of alpha-adrenoceptor

Patients should let their doctor know if they have any prostate problems, as midodrine may worsen symptoms. Common side effects of midodrine are urinary retention, frequent urination, chills, and tingling of the scalp. Anxiety, nervousness, dry mouth, and head pain are less common.

Beta-Blockers

Beta-blockers work to slow down heart rate and lower blood pressure. Common side effects of lowered blood pressure are dizziness and fatigue. It's important for patients to let their physician know if they experience these symptoms or find them bothersome. Patients should report to their physician right away if they experience a slow pulse, which is defined as less than 60 beats per minute. A lower dose may be needed. Common side effects are difficulty sleeping, drowsiness, decreased sex drive, nervousness, depression, nightmares, upset stomach, constipation, and diarrhea. Patients with coexisting mast cell activation disorders may want to use beta-blockers with caution, as this type of drug can cause degranulation of mast cells, which may worsen symptoms.

Clonidine (Catapres®) lowers blood pressure in a different way than beta-blockers. It does this by decreasing the circulating amount of the norepinephrine in the blood. Norepinephrine is one of the chemical messengers responsible for stimulating the sympathetic nervous system. Clonidine creates a blockade to help prevent this messenger from getting released. Clonidine can also be used to help patients withdraw from addictive substances. Side effects of clonidine can include drowsiness, dry mouth, dizziness, and constipation.

Yohimbine, unlike Clonidine, increases blood pressure. While it blocks the same receptors that clonidine activates, yohimbine actually releases more norepinephrine into the bloodstream. Norepinephrine is one of the chemicals responsible for stimulating the sympathetic nervous system, raising blood pressure. Common side effects of yohimbine are trembling, paleness of skin, goosebumps, hair standing out, increased salivation, and emotional changes.

Amphetamines or **Methylphenidate**, are often recognizable as ADHD medication. These stimulants help push norepinephrine where it needs to go, thus making it more effective. These help blood vessels

failure to properly tighten blood vessels. This is very effective for increasing blood pressure in patients with orthostatic intolerance and orthostatic hypotension. Midodrine is one of only a few drugs approved by the FDA for orthostatic hypotension and other forms of dysautonomia.

Midodrine can cause hypertension, which can be especially exaggerated when the patient is supine. Midodrine can also worsen symptoms of prostate problems, such as urinary retention, urgency, and decreased urinary stream. Alpha-1 adrenoceptor blockers used for treating benign prostatic hypertrophy can interfere with midodrine.[5] Side effects of midodrine are mostly due to the action on alpha-adrenergic receptors of the hair follicles, causing chills and tingling.

Beta-Blockers

Beta-blockers help to decrease heart rate and blood pressure. Beta-blockers have been shown to help chronic headaches in dysautonomia patients. It is important to pay attention to blood pressure, as many dysautonomia patients often experience hypotension. This hypotensive response can be exaggerated after a dose of beta-blockers. Patients may complain of worsened fatigue while on beta-blockers. Beta-blockers are not a mainstay for patients with mast cell activation disorders, as they are known to cause mast cell degranulation, which often exacerbates symptoms in this cohort of patients. Beta-blockers can also reduce plasma renin activity, which has been correlated with hypovolemic states.[6] Beta-blockers should be given in low doses.

Non-Selective beta-blockers, such as Propranolol®, are helpful in patients who have high epinephrine levels, such as those with hyperadrenergic hypertension. Since non-selective beta-blockers block both beta-1 and beta-2 receptors, they therefore will help to block the effects of epinephrine at the receptor.

Selective beta-blockers, such as Metoprolol®, are more useful in primary POTS and dysautonomias that do not present with increased epinephrine levels. It is important to figure out whether associated tachycardia is a primary or compensatory response. If tachycardia is a compensatory response for a hypovolemic state, then beta-blockers will not be of much help. Beta-blockers often work well patients that have tachycardia as a primary response.

tighten, raise blood pressure, increase attention span, decrease appetite, and lessen fatigue. Stimulants must be used with caution, however, because there is a risk for the body to become dependent on them. Weight loss and insomnia are the two most common side effects of these stimulants.

Droxidopa (Northera®)

Droxidopa, is a synthetic amino acid that works as a "pre-drug" to increase norepinephrine in the body. Droxidopa was recently approved by the FDA for use in patients with neurogenic orthostatic hypotension (NOH), multiple symptom atrophy (MSA), pure autonomic failure (PAF) and Parkinson's disease (PD). With over 20 years on the market, relatively few patients report side effects, including tachycardia, hypertension, nausea, vomiting, and headache.

Selective Serotonin Reuptake Inhibitors (SSRIs) medications are often used to treat depression and anxiety. They are sometimes helpful with complications often associated with dysautonomia. Conditions like hyper visceral sensitivity and irritable bowel syndrome are commonly treated with these medications. Side effects of SSRI medications may include changes in mood, weight gain, difficulty falling asleep, headache, reduced sexual drive, and dizziness. Great care must be taken to report any changes in behavior, especially in the first few days of use as these medications have the potential to cause depression. Suicide risk is increased while on this medication, especially in teens.

Benzodiazepines are medications such as Xanax® and Klonopin®. They are often used to treat anxiety and panic attacks. Sometimes they are used to treat nausea and vomiting. Klonopin®, unlike other benzodiazepines, also helps multiple system atrophy patients with sleep difficulties[1], and reduces palpitations and oscillations in blood flow[2]. They are addictive and should be used with caution as stopping them suddenly may cause seizures and death. Common side effects include drowsiness, dizziness, and headache. Mental changes can occur, like irritability, depression, memory loss, or unclear thinking.

Clonidine (Catapres®) stimulates alpha-2 adrenoceptors and decreases overall sympathetic nervous system tone. It works to suppress the amount of norepinephrine released. This suppression leads to a decrease in blood pressure. Patients with long-term hypertension can benefit from this drug, such as those in hyperadrenergic states. Clonidine's sedative properties can limit its usage.

Yohimbine, blocks alpha-2 adrenoceptors that clonidine activates. This medication, however, dumps norepinephrine into the blood vessels where it binds with alpha-1 adrenoceptors. Yohimbine has been shown to increase plasma norepinephrine levels. This causes an increase in blood pressure. Dysautonomia patients with chronic autonomic failure, multiple system atrophy, and autonomically mediated syncope may benefit from this drug.

Amphetamines or **Methylphenidate**, when used with caution, can be very helpful in improving the function of patients with chronic orthostatic intolerance. A powerful vasoconstrictor, these stimulants also help to increase attention span and lessen fatigue. There is a potential for tolerance and dependence. Extreme caution should be used with underweight patients or patients at risk of malnutrition.

Droxidopa (Northera®)

Droxidopa, also known as L-DOPS, L-Dihydroxyphenylserine, is a synthetic amino acid that is helpful for patients with neurogenic orthostatic hypotension (NOH) and other forms of autonomic failure. It is very closely related chemically to L-dihydroxyphenylalanine (Levodopa, L-DOPA), which is an effective drug to treat Parkinson's disease. L-DOPA works by being converted in the brain to the catecholamine, dopamine. Although L-DOPS crosses the blood-brain barrier, it works by being converted to the closely related catecholamine, norepinephrine, mainly outside the brain increasing peripheral circulating epinephrine and norepinephrine. Droxidopa was recently approved by the US FDA for dysautonomia patients with autonomic failure.

Selective Serotonin Reuptake Inhibitors (SSRIs) are considered second generation antidepressants, after tricyclic antidepressants (TCAs)

Intravenous Saline

IV therapy has been shown to be useful in patients with POTS and other forms of dysautonomia that include dizziness and fatigue. It works to increase the fluid volume in the body, which raises blood pressure and lessens the workload of the heart. It has also been found to be beneficial for temporarily combating fatigue, improving gastric motility, and helping with headaches. Routine IV infusions can be a hassle. An infusion usually requires home health care or a trip to a local infusion center. Repeated needles sticks to the veins can cause trauma, so a device such as a port or permanent central line may need to be used. These can be bothersome to the patient and are not recommended in most patients due to the increased the risk for infection.

---

[1] Ferini-Strambi L. et al. "Sleep Dysfunction in Multiple System Atrophy" Curr Treat Options Neurol. 2012. Milan, Italy. Oct;14(5):464-73

[2] Thompson, Charles R. Interview. Pensacola, FL; December, 2011.

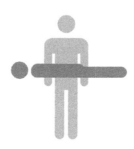

and monoamine oxidase inhibitors (MAOIs), and are used primarily for treatment in major depressive disorder and other mood disorders. These medications may be helpful with treating dysautonomia patients with comorbid conditions or complications. SSRI medications can be used to treat the dysautonomia patient experiencing chronic depression or anxiety. They are also commonly used to treat conditions like hyper visceral sensitivity and irritable bowel syndrome. Neurotransmitters such as norepinephrine, dopamine, adrenaline, serotonin, and acetylcholine are often released abnormally in patients with POTS and can affect the mental state of the POTS patient. (It should be noted that SNRIs are not recommended for POTS patients as norepinephrine reuptake inhibitors have been found to worsen symptoms.[7])

Extreme caution should be used with SSRIs, especially in teenagers and children. Low doses should be initiated at first and the patient monitored closely, especially in the first few days, for signs of depression or suicidal ideation.

Benzodiazapines such as clonazepam (Klonopin®) can be very helpful in improving REM sleep in patients with multiple system atrophy[8] (MSA) and other forms of dysautonomia where sleep disturbances are seen. Additionally, clonazepam is thought to decrease palpitations and oscillations of blood flow by blunting adrenergic stimulation and reducing syncope. Other benzodiazepines such as Alprazolam (Xanax) can be used to help relax the mood in patients with prominent anxiety, panic attacks, nausea, and vomiting. Due to their highly addictive nature, caution should be taken when prescribing benzodiazapines.

Intravenous Saline

IV therapy increases circulating blood volume and helps with hypervolemia symptoms sometimes seen in patients with postural orthostatic tachycardia syndrome, as well as other dysautonomias. IV infusions help decrease palpitations, raise blood pressure, lessen orthostatic tachycardia, help with fatigue, improve migraines, and increase gastrointestinal motility in some patients. Patients with gastroparesis often find it difficult to consume the daily-recommended amount of water. Excessive water intake can also lead to shifts in electrolyte balance, whereas an IV infusion provides isotonic hydration.[9]

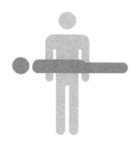

Although there is anecdotal evidence that 1 liter of IV saline given over a period of one hour improves symptoms in POTS patients for up to 48 hours[10], caution must be used in prescribing infusions as fluid overload can lead to hypervolemia, which can result in life threatening conditions such as heart failure and pulmonary edema.[11]

In some cases where regular infusions are needed, a power port or permanent central line may be considered, but the decision to use should be balanced with the risk of infection.

[1] National Dysautonomia Research Foundation.

[2] Palma, J.-A., Kaufmann, L., Fuente, C., Percival, L., Mendoza, C., & Kaufmann, H. (2014). Current Treatments in Familial Dysautonomia. Expert Opinion on Pharmacotherapy, 15(18), 2653–2671. doi:10.1517/14656566.2014.970530.

[3] Thompson, Charles R. Interview. Pensacola, Florida; December, 2011.

[4] Raj, Satish. Expert Opinion. August, 2015.

[5] National Dysautonomia Research Foundation.

[6] Neurological disorders. (n.d.). Retrieved June 14, 2015, from *http://www.med help.org/tags/health_page/39830/neurological-disorders/Dysautonomia-Treat ments?hp_id=171.*

[7] Green, Elizabeth et al. "Effects of Norepinephrine Reuptake Inhibition on Postural Tachycardia Syndrome" J Am Heart Assoc. 2013;2:eOOO395.

[8] Ferini-Strambi L. et al. "Sleep Dysfunction in Multiple System Atrophy" Curr Treat Options Neurol. 2012. Milan, Italy. Oct;14(5):464-73.

[9] Thompson, Charles R. Interview. Pensacola, Florida; December, 2011.

[10] Santa Maria, R. (2013, April 1). Saline Therapy: Hydration Found to Be a Powerful Tool in Treatment of Dysautonomia (POTS). Retrieved June 14, 2015, from *http://santamariamedicine.com/2013/04/saline-therapy-hydration-found-to-be-a-powerful-tool-in-treatment-of-dysautonomia-pots/.*

[11] Sheldon, Robert et al. "2015 Heart Rhythm Society Expert Concensus Statement on the Diagnosis and treatment of Postural Tachycardia Syndrome, Inappropriate Sinus Tachycardia, and Vasovagal Syncope." May 13, 2015.

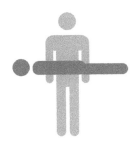

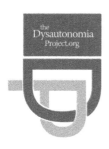

33

TOP 20 DYSAUTONOMIA DRUGS*

Several drug treatments are used for dysautonomias. Some of them are powerful or can produce harmful side effects. Patients should take medications only under the supervision of a doctor with expertise and experience in the treatment of dysautonomias.

Drug Name / Class	Helps with	Notes
Fludrocortisone (Florinef®)	Increases blood volume and blood pressure. May help in reducing plasma NE with long-term use. (Orthostatic intolerance and orthostatic hypotension.)	Increase dietary sodium for maximum effectiveness. Ideal in low doses.
Midodrine (Proamatine®)	Tightens blood vessels, increases blood pressure and prevents fainting. (Orthostatic hypotension, POTS and other forms of dysautonomia.)	Can cause supine hypertension.
Beta-Blocker	Decrease heart rate, blood pressure and adrenaline effects. Prevents fainting. (POTS and hyperadrenergic hypertension.)	Known to cause mast cell degranulation.
Pyridostigmine (Mestinon®)	Increases blood pressure and muscle strength. Reduces breakdown of Acetylcholine in ANS. (Chronic orthostatic intolerance.)	
IV Saline	Increase in blood volume, orthostatic tolerance and cognitive function. (POTS and orthostatic hypotension)	Symptom improvement is temporary. Caution should be used when prescribing.
Clonidine (Catapres®) or Methyldopa (Aldomet®)	Decreases blood pressure and hyperadrenergic responses. Also improves sleep. Decreases sympathetic adrenergic stimulation.	
Amphetamine (Adderall®) Or Methylphenidate (Ritalin®, Concerta®)	Tighten blood vessels. Increases alertness, cognitive function, and improves brain fog. Reduces appetite. (Chronic orthostatic intolerance)	Use with caution as can be addictive.
Ibuprofen (Motrin®)	Tighten blood vessels. Blocks inflammatory prostaglandins.	

Clonazepam (Klonopin®)	Regulate oscillations of blood flow to heart and vital organs and increased sense of calmness. (Multiple system atrophy and chronic orthostatic intolerance.)	Recommended start with low dose at bedtime.
Alprazolam (Xanax®)	Increase sense of calmness.	Sedative effect.
Droxidopa (Northera®) Also known as L-DOPS	Increase blood pressure. (Neurogenic orthostatic hypotension and other forms of autonomic failure.)	One of the few FDA approved drugs for neurogenic Orthostatic Hypotension.
Tricyclic Antidepressants (E.g. Doxepin)	Improve mood.	
Selective Serotonin Reuptake Inhibitor, (SSRIs)	Improves mood, reduces anxiety.	May cause depression – use caution with teens.
Erythropoietin (Procrit®)	Increase blood count and blood pressure. Especially helpful with anemic patients or patients with chronic fatigue.	Difficult to gain coverage through insurance.
Yohimbine	Increase blood pressure (Chronic autonomic failure, multiple system atrophy and autonomically mediated sycope.)	
Ivabradine (Corlanor®)	Reduces heart rate, angina pectoris, and improves inappropriate sinus tachycardia (IST).	Useful for patients unable to tolerate beta-blockers.
Somatostatin (Octreotide®)	Tighten blood vessels in gut.	
Desmopressin (DDAVP®) "	Tighten blood vessels and causes kidneys to retain water	
Bethanechol (=Urecholine®)	Increase salivation, gut action, and urination.	
H1 & H2 Antihistamines	Tightens blood vessels. Improves inflammation of the gut.	May be helpful in patients with coexisting mast cell activation.

This top 20 list may change based on feedback of The Dysautonomia Project members and advisors. Check our website for the most updated top 20 list at: www.TheDysautonomiaProject.org/Resources/8.

34

MANAGING PAIN

HOW DO I LIVE WITH THIS PAIN

by Pradeep Chopra, MD

Chronic pain in patients with dysautonomia is usually due to an underlying cause. For example, a patient with neuropathy (pain due to nerve damage) may develop dysautonomia. The pain in this case is because of the neuropathy and not the dysautonomia. Dysautonomia may make it more challenging for the patient to function. Patients with certain coexisting conditions are more prone to chronic pain in dysautonomia, such as those with Ehlers Danlos syndrome, complex regional pain syndrome, fibromyalgia, and other chronic neuropathic pain conditions.

The main symptoms of dysautonomia are feeling lightheaded, fainting or almost fainting, headaches, blurry vision, fatigue, poor concentration, palpitations, nausea and vomiting, unable to do low impact exercises, shortness of breath and air hunger.

> For therapy and medications, start low and go slow.

Patients who are disabled for several months from chronic pain are more prone to developing symptoms of orthostatic intolerance (a form or dysautonomia)[1]. In a study done at the Mayo Clinic in patients with dysautonomia, 74% had fatigue, and 88% had chronic pain (chronic headache in 69% and chronic abdominal pain in 39%).[2]

Fatigue is much more common in adolescents. When patients have a difficult time functioning because of their pain, their symptoms of dysautonomia also worsen and make them even more disabled. Both conditions should be treated at the same time.

34

MANAGING PAIN

IN PATIENTS WITH DYSAUTONOMIA

by Pradeep Chopra, MD

Pain may be nociceptive (structural) pain or neuropathic pain. Chronic pain has an element of both nociceptive pain and neuropathic pain. Some conditions may have one more than the other. For example, in osteoarthritis the pain is predominantly nociceptive, but there is also some pain that is neuropathic. Diabetic neuropathy has some nociceptive pain.

Dysautonomia is much more common in neuropathic pain conditions, such as complex regional pain syndrome (also known as reflex sympathetic dystrophy). Conditions that are commonly associated with dysautonomia are Ehlers Danlos syndrome (EDS), complex regional pain syndrome (CRPS), fibromyalgia, migraines and chronic daily headaches.

> *Managing pain should be directed towards restoring function.*

Patients with chronic pain and dysautonomia have a dual set of issues. Patients may be non-functional because of their chronic pain and orthostatic intolerance. Ideally both of these problems should be managed at the same time. Fatigue is a symptom of orthostatic intolerance. Fatigue is also associated with chronic pain. Managing fatigue will depend on optimal pain control and managing the patient's symptoms of orthostatic intolerance. Treating one without the other will be challenging.

One of the challenges in treating this population of patients is the perceived behavioral aspect. Conditions such as EDS, CRPS and fibromyalgia are common in adolescent to young females. A classical presentation

Neuropathic pain (pain due to damaged nerves) is common in chronic pain. Neuropathy may happen in peripheral nerves, but it can also affect autonomic nerves (nerves that control automatic functions in the body, such as heart beating, blood pressure, movement of intestines). Once neuropathic pain affects the autonomic nervous system, it presents with symptoms of dysautonomia.

Common Patient Complaints

- *I get pain in the back of my neck and head. You know, it's an ache that comes and goes, usually with stress, in that region around my neck and shoulders.*

- *When my symptoms flare up I can't get out of bed and my body hurts all over. It is hard to explain.*

- *I have pain all over. I can't think of a place in my body where I'm not experiencing pain. Ok, maybe my earlobes.*

- *My right leg always hurts. It's a dull ache. Some days it is worse than others.*

- *I have horrible migraine headaches almost every day. Usually on a scale of 6-9 out of 10.*

- *I have these very sharp pains in my chest. Sometimes they are like a stabbing pain. Sometimes they are a burning pain. No one can tell me why I get them.*

Most patients do not relate their symptoms of pain to their symptoms of dysautonomia. They do not mention their pain to their cardiologist or neurologist who is treating their dysautonomia. On the other hand, patients do not mention their symptoms of dizziness and palpitations to their pain medicine specialist.

Tips for Managing Pain in Dysautonomia:

1. Hydrate well. Drink plenty of fluids with electrolytes. Sports drinks are good for hydrating. Hydrating improves symptoms of dysautonomia and muscle spasms.

2. Exercise releases natural pain-relieving chemicals in the system. Exercise in some form every day should be a part of every patient's treatment plan. Exercise helps improve function and helps blood flow, which prevents stiffness.

is severe disabling pain, syncope, pre-syncope, fatigue, headaches, and nausea. Physicians who are not aware of the connection between chronic pain and dysautonomia often brand these patients with a behavioral diagnosis. This, in turn, is devastating for the patient because all avenues of treating the real condition are closed. Understandably, these young patients with a severe condition may have an element of depression, but the correct management lies in treating the underlying organic condition.

> *Central Sensitization is the key to explaining chronic pain. Treatment goals must include decreasing central sensitization and restoring function.*

Treatment options are directed toward restoring function rather than focused on lowering pain. It is very important that a multidisciplinary approach be taken that includes a pain medicine specialist, cardiologist, physical therapist, and an occupational therapist. Treatment should start with eliciting a good history and performing a physical examination rather than relying purely on imaging studies or laboratory tests. Once the underlying issues are identified, they should be approached by specialists working together with the goal of restoring function.

Pradeep Chopra, MD, MHCM is a Pain Medicine specialist with a special interest in complex pain conditions such as Ehlers Danlos Syndrome and Complex Regional Pain Syndrome in adults and children. Dr. Chopra completed his residency in Anesthesia and Critical Care from Harvard Medical School. He completed his Fellowship in Pain Medicine from Harvard Medical School. He is now an Assistant Professor (Clinical) at Brown Medical School, Rhode Island, USA, and the Director, Multidisciplinary Pain Management Center. He is the recipient of many awards, including The Schwartz Center Compassionate Caregiver Award 2013.

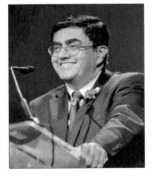

3. Use Narcotics sparingly: Narcotics in high doses, or taken for prolonged periods of time, may sensitize you to pain, forcing you to take more which, in turn, sensitizes you to pain even more, especially in neuropathic pain. Short courses of small dose narcotics may be helpful, if they help you exercise more, which is far more beneficial in the long run.

4. Discuss your pain with your doctor. If appropriate, seek the advice of pain experts who consult with your primary care physician and specialists who treat your dysautonomia.

5. Consider pain when you sleep. Pain may prevent you from sleeping. If you take a sedative, then the pain keeps you awake and the sedative makes you groggy, making things worse. If the pain keeps you awake, then consider measures to treat pain rather than taking a sedative. Follow the rules of good sleep hygiene. Discuss this with your doctor.

6. Develop an arsenal of "pain-helpers." Ideas include cool compresses, stretching techniques, vitamin C, comfortable clothes, well-fitting shoes, good sleep hygiene.

---

[1] Mack KJ, Johnson JN, Rowe P: Orthostatic Intolerance and the headache patient. Semin Pediatr Neurol 17:109-116. 2010. Elsevier.

[2] Fischer PR, Brands CK, Porter CJ et al: High prevalence of orthostatic intolerance in adolescents in a General Pediatric Referral Clinic. Clin Autonom Res 15:340, 2005

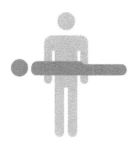

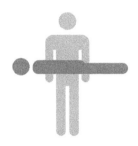

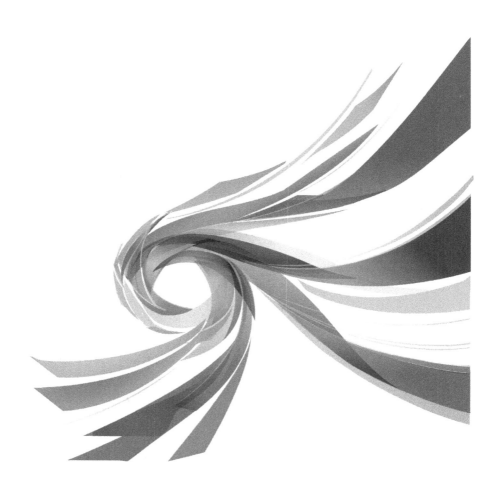

SECTION 6

JOIN
THE DYSAUTONOMIA PROJECT

COLLABORATE WITH MANY PHYSICIANS AND PATIENTS TO TRANSFORM HOW DYSAUTONOMIA IS TREATED IN YOUR COMMUNITY.

If you want to go fast go alone.
If you want to go far, go together.

African Proverb

35

NEXT STEPS

How You Can Be Part
of the Dysautonomia Project

This book is a starting point for bridging the knowledge gap between decades of research in autonomic medicine and that of patients, community-based physicians, and other health care practitioners. It is not a "how-to" book written by one person, one doctor, or by a group of doctors, but the collaborative effort of many physicians and patients from many parts of the world who are working together to speed the time to diagnosis of dysautonomias and transform the patient physician interaction through education and meaningful dialogue at the community level.

From this starting point, which is an introduction to dysautonomia, there are many next steps for learning. Next steps for patients include:

- Share information in this book with your local physicians(s) and others and/or buy an extra copy of the book and give it to your favorite doctor as a present.

- Grow in your knowledge of your specific case, including working together with your physician(s) in developing a treatment plan based on good information so you can improve your health.

- Become an advocate for your case.

- Access more in-depth information via online learning and the resources found at *www.TheDysautonomiaProject.org/resources*.

- Join The Dysautonomia Project as a free member by visiting *www.thedysautonomiaproject.org*.

- Like us on our facebook page to stay current on new information.

35

NEXT STEPS

JOIN THE DYSAUTONOMIA PROJECT

This book is a starting point for bridging the knowledge gap between decades of research in the area of autonomic medicine and that of community-based physicians and other health care practitioners. It is not a "how-to" book written by one doctor or a group of doctors, but the collaborative effort of many physicians and patients working together to speed the time to diagnosis of dysautonomias and transform the patient physician interaction through education and meaningful dialogue.

From this starting point, which is an introduction to dysautonomia, there are many next steps for learning. Next steps for physicians include:

- Participate in The Dysautonomia Project's 1-hour Grand Rounds CME program that looks at 5 heterogeneous case studies.

- Share information in this book with your patients, other physicians, and community leaders in your area.

- Read "Principles of Autonomic Medicine," a free online medical text by co-author David S. Goldstein, MD, PhD. This book is available at: *www.TheDysautonomiaProject.org/resources/2* free of charge.

- Grow in your practice of autonomic medicine, including making efforts to "flip the clinic" as discussed in chapter 25.

- Access more in-depth information about autonomic medicine online, including resources found at *www.TheDysautonomiaProject.org/resources*.

- Contact us if you would like to be a part of The Dysautonomia Project activities in your local area.

As in all medicine, the evaluation and management of patients is not an exact science but a practice that changes and improves with time, research, and quality education. The Dysautonomia Project members and advisors collaborate for continuous improvement of all aspects of the educational materials including:

- Dysautonomia Clinical Assessment Form
- Protocol for Conducting Orthostatic Vitals Test
- Top 20 Drug List
- Top 10 Non-Pharmacological Treatments
- Physician List
- Content of The Dysautonomia Project Book
- Content of The Dysautonomia Project Website
- Content of The Dysautonomia Project Grand Rounds CME

If you are a member (you can join for free online) or advisor and would like to make a suggestion for improvement, please submit the continuous improvement form found at:

www.TheDysautonomiaProject.org/resources/9.

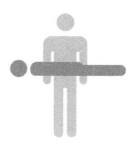

- Consider a certificate program in autonomic medicine offered by the United Council for Neurologic Subspecialties. For more information visit *https://www.ucns.org/go/subspecialty/autonomic/certification.*
- Join The Dysautonomia Project as a free member by visiting *www.thedysautonomiaproject.org.*
- Contact us if you would like to be added to our physician list.
- Send us an email at *info@TheDysautonomiaProject.org* if you want to be considered as a medical advisor for The Dysautonomia Project activities in your local area. (This involves being a resource for medical questions and/or participating in select activities for physicians in your area.)

As in all medicine, the evaluation and management of patients is not an exact science but a practice that changes and improves with time, research, and quality education. The Dysautonomia Project members and advisors collaborate for continuous improvement of all aspects of the educational materials available.

If you are a member (you can join for free online) and would like to make a suggestion for improvement, please submit the continuous improvement form found at

www.TheDysautonomiaProject.org/resources/9.

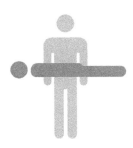

36

ABOUT THE DYSAUTONOMIA PROJECT

The Dysautonomia Project is a 501(c)(3) not-for-profit organization aimed at using education to bridge the wide knowledge gap between decades of scientific research and that of community based health care providers. Educational efforts center on primary educational offerings:

- The Dysautonomia Project Book: This is an introduction to autonomic nervous system disorders for physicians and patients.

- The Dysautonomia Project Website: A central site to access resources for greater understanding. It includes videos and tools for physicians and patients.

- The Dysautonomia Project 1-hour Grand Rounds CME Course: An introductory course for physicians that utilizes the book as the core text and features five heterogeneous case studies.

The project launched in the metropolitan area of Tampa Bay, Florida in October, 2014, and is currently expanding into communities across the nation and the world.

This book is a starting point for collaboration among:

- Expert physicians of autonomic medicine and related research,

- Local physicians who frequently have no formal training in autonomic medicine,

- Community leaders and the general public, and

- Patients/family members who have suffered while waiting an average of 6 years for a diagnosis.

Mission

To create awareness and raise funds for education of the medical community, healthcare providers, and the general population about dysautonomia (disorders of the autonomic [automatic] nervous system).

The Big Goal

The big goal is to train an interdisciplinary team of local physicians in every major community in the United States in the next decade. Although physicians may not become experts in autonomic medicine, they would be able to provide basic autonomic assessment and treatment in consultation with experts in the field, such as The Dysautonomia Project's contributing authors, medical advisors, and other specialists of autonomic medicine.

10-Year Vision

To collaborate with patients, physicians, health care provides, hospitals, as well as local, state, and national leaders, to provide easy-to-access and easy-to-understand education about disorders of the autonomic nervous system (ANS) based on more than 30 years of clinical data from leading dysautonomia researchers around the world. By achieving this vision we would:

- Reduce health care costs by eliminating unnecessary physician visits, diagnostic tests, and patient services. Serve as a model in the area of introductory dysautonomia education for physicians around the world.
- Strive to make "dysautonomia" a household word.

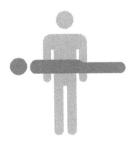

37

WE NEED YOUR HELP

The Dysautonomia Project, a not-for-profit organization, is run completely by volunteers. To really make a difference, we need an enormous team of volunteers. Today we need help in the following areas:

- **Donations:** For the production and publication of educational materials, programs, and the achievement of our mission. To make an online donation, visit *www.TheDysautonomiaProject.org.*

- **Volunteers:** We have an army of volunteers behind the scenes who work to keep The Dysautonomia Project running and growing. We have many needs, from leading activities in your community, to planning and producing patient education videos for the website, to addressing envelopes for special events.

- **Creating Awareness:** Join as a free member online at *www.TheDysautonomiaProject.org* to learn more about what you can do to help spread the word in your community.

- **Buy this book for your physician(s).** Tell us about it and consider adding your physician to our growing list of physicians who know about dysautonomias. If added, the physicians may be included in periodic medical education updates. All proceeds from the sale of this book go toward supporting the mission of The Dysautonomia Project.

Consider sharing your time, talents and/or treasures. Together we can create hope for the future.

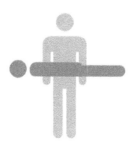

APPENDICES

APPENDIX A

DYSAUTONOMIA CLINICAL ASSESSEMENT FORM

This form is designed for physicians and/or nurse practitioners to use as a guide in clinical assessment of autonomic nervous system function. Page one includes sample questions and notes. Page two is blank. Extra copies may be downloaded from *www.TheDysautonomiaProject.org/Resources/10.*

Chief Complaint	In a few words, what is the main problem bothering you that brings you here today?
History of Present Illness	When was the last time you felt completely healthy? What was the first thing that went wrong? What happened next? Have you noticed anything that makes the problem worse or better? What treatments have been tried, and how did you respond? (Note: These questions only cover some aspects of autonomic screening.)
Autonomic Review of Systems	Who does your shopping? Are you able to tolerate standing, exercise, heat, a large meal? Do you sweat like other people? Do you make spit like other people? Have you noticed any problems with urination? Have you noticed any problems with bowel movements? Have you noticed any problems with sexual function?
Prescribed or OTC Medications and Supplements	(Make note of any which may affect hemodynamics and/or main chemical messengers of the ANS such as NE, EPI, and/or Ach.)
Past Hx	
Family Hx	
Personal and Social Hx	
Physical Exam	Water bottle sign? Signs of pooling of blood in feet? Cyanosis, dependent edema?
Orthostatic Vitals Test	Normal / Abnormal?

Chief Complaint	
History of Present Illness	
Autonomic Review of Systems	
Prescribed or OTC Medications and Supplements	
Past Hx	
Family Hx	
Personal and Social Hx	
Physical Exam	
Orthostatic Vitals Test	Normal / Abnormal?

APPENDIX B

Protocol for Conducting an Orthostatic Vitals Test

Aim

Physicians and/or nurse practitioners measure orthostatic vitals in conjunction with a comprehensive clinical assessment. Orthostatic Vitals are an important initial measure in the assessment of patients with dysautonomia, a group of disorders of the autonomic nervous system. This test may be conducted in the clinic or hospital setting and may help the physician in patient assessment. Physicians, clinic or hospital staff, and/or other trained health care professionals may use this protocol. A video demonstration of this procedure is available for viewing at *www.TheDysautonomiaProject.org/Resources/11.*

Requirements

The test lasts approximately 15 minutes, is non-invasive, and requires the use of:

- A blood pressure cuff
- Capability to measure the patient's heart rate (e.g., palpating pulse, or pulse oximeter)
- A clock or stopwatch
- A bed or exam table that is low enough to the ground that the patient can sit on the edge of the table with feet resting on the floor
- A copy of the Orthostatic Vitals Test Form (see attached)
- A quiet room

Due to the diurnal variability of hemodynamics, it is ideal to conduct this test in the morning hours, but it may be conducted any time during the day.

Before the Test

Before the test it is important to explain the test procedure to the patient, including:

- Length of procedure
- Use of blood pressure cuff and heart rate monitoring
- Importance of not speaking during the test unless answering a question
- Goal of the first 5-10 minutes of the test is to be as relaxed as possible. No use of cell phone, reading, etc. is permitted.

Conducting the Orthostatic Vitals Test

1. Resting Phase = 5 to 10 minutes: The goal for this phase is to establish a baseline resting heart rate. Have the patient lie down with both legs fully extended (not crossed) for at least five minutes. (If you have time, 10 minutes is optimal for relaxation.) At the beginning of this phase place the blood pressure cuff and heart rate monitor, if appropriate. At the end of the resting phase measure the patient's resting heart rate. It is ideal to palpate the pulse for 1 minute average heart rate or (30 sec x2). At the end of the resting phase take a baseline resting blood pressure and ask the patient, "How do you feel right now?" If they report that they feel fine record "no symptoms." Record the results of the resting blood pressure and resting heart rate. Transition: Before transitioning to the sitting phase tell the patient that you are about to ask them to sit up for a few minutes but, before they do, it is important they sit upright as much as possible at the edge of the bed or exam table with feet resting on the floor without leaning back on anything or moving their body and, if possible, without supporting their weight on their hands.

2. Sitting Phase = 2 minutes: Observe to ensure patient is seated properly with both feet on the ground. After the patient is seated properly, ask, "How are you feeling now?" Record any reported symptoms. After two minutes take the

patient's heart rate and blood pressure. Record the results before transitioning to the standing phase. Transition: Before transitioning to the standing phase tell the patient that you are about to have them stand up for up to five minutes. As in the resting and sitting phase, you will be asking them how they feel. If at anytime during this portion of the test they begin to feel faint they should sit down immediately. They should not ask for permission to sit because we want to make sure they are safe and avoid any possibility of fainting. Emphasize that their safety is more important than this test and that it is not a problem if they do not finish the entire test. Also explain that when they stand it is important to stand as still as possible and not lean on the bed or exam table. Tell them you will be taking their heart rate and blood pressure at 1, 3 and 5 minutes. Ask if they have any questions.

3. Standing Phase = 5 minutes: Observe to ensure patient is standing properly with both feet on the floor. After the patient is standing, ask, "How are you feeling now?" Record any reported symptoms. After one minute take the patient's heart rate and blood pressure and record. Do the same thing at 3 minutes and 5 minutes. Record the observations. Once all answers are recorded ask the patient to sit down, or lie down if that would feel more comfortable.

    IMPORTANT: If at any time the patient reports feeling faint or lightheaded ask them if they want to sit down and end the test. Remind them there is no problem if the test is ended early. If the test ends early record as much information as you have been able to collect during the time of the test, as well as the time in which the test stopped.

4. Recovery: While the patient is sitting or lying down complete the summary information on the form.

Reported symptoms are of equal importance as recorded quantifiable data; therefore what the patient says should be documented. When possible use quotations to document actual phrases used. If necessary, ask questions to clarify what the patient means. For instance, if the patient says, "I'm feeling dizzy," it may be helpful to clarify if that is a symptom of vertigo (a sensation of spinning) or a symptom of presyncope (a prodromal feeling of faintness). If there is not enough room inside the table, use the margin or even back side of the page for recording reported symptoms.

(See Orthostatics Vital Test Form on following two pages.)

Orthostatic Vitals Test Form		
Before the Test	**Explanation of Procedure** - Use of blood pressure cuff and heart rate measurement - Important not to speak unless answering a question - Goal, first 5-10 minutes: to be as relaxed as possible (no phone, reading, etc.) - Explain why we do the test	
1. Resting Phase= 5-10 minutes	Ensure proper position with feet extended.	
Notes:	Resting Supine HR:	Supine BP:
	Reported Symptoms:	
	Transition: Explain before sitting - Sit upright as much as possible at the edge, feet on floor - Avoid leaning, moving their body and, if possible, without supporting weight with hands.	
2. Sitting Phase= 2 minutes	Ensure proper position.	
Notes:	Sitting HR:	Sitting BP:
	Reported Symptoms:	
	Transition: Explain before standing -Stand for up to five minutes. -If at anytime they begin to feel faint, sit down immediately. (Do not ask to sit because their safety is most important.) - It is not a problem if they do not finish the entire test. - It is important to stand as still as possible, avoid leaning.	

3. Standing Phase= 5 minutes	Ensure proper position.	
Notes:	1 Minute Standing HR:	1 Minute Standing BP:
	Reported Symptoms:	
	3 Minute Standing HR:	3 Minute Standing BP:
	Reported Symptoms:	
	5 Minute Standing HR:	5 Minute Standing BP:
	Reported Symptoms:	
	Explain that the test is done. They can either sit or lie down during the next few minutes to rest.	

Summary

Resting HR _____ **Resting BP** _____

Sitting HR _____ **Sitting BP** _____

Standing HR 1 _____ **Standing BP 1**_____

Standing HR 3 _____ **Standing BP 3**_____

Standing HR 5_____ **Standing BP 5**_____

Orthostatic HR Increase:_____ bpm   (difference between resting & highest standing HR)

Do you want to bring The Dysautonomia Project
to your community?
Send us and email message at
info@TheDysautonomiaProject.org.

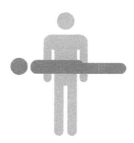

Printed in the USA
CPSIA information can be obtained
at www.ICGtesting.com
LVHW040413270724
786603LV00001B/201